T0263240

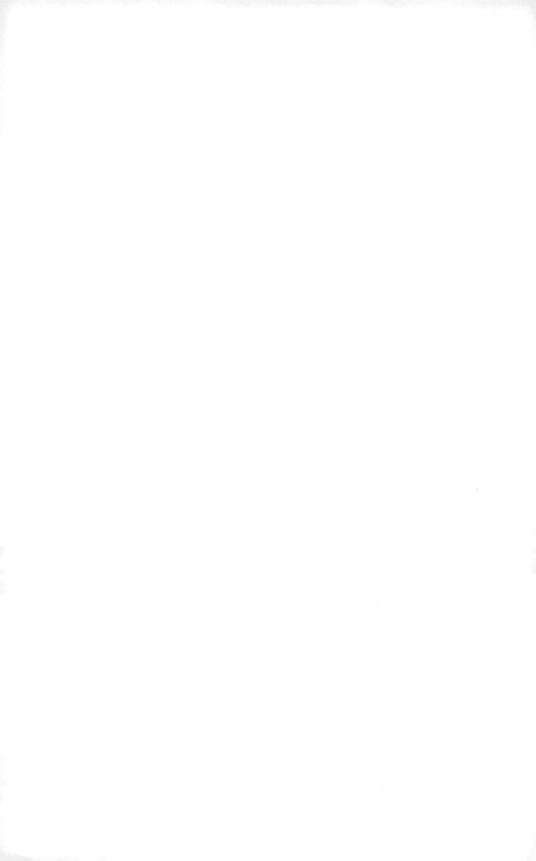

Infections and Asthma

Editor

MITCHELL H. GRAYSON

IMMUNOLOGY AND ALLERGY CLINICS OF NORTH AMERICA

www.immunology.theclinics.com

Consulting Editor
STEPHEN A. TILLES

August 2019 • Volume 39 • Number 3

ELSEVIER

1600 John F. Kennedy Boulevard • Suite 1800 • Philadelphia, Pennsylvania, 19103-2899

http://www.theclinics.com

IMMUNOLOGY AND ALLERGY CLINICS OF NORTH AMERICA Volume 39, Number 3

August 2019 ISSN 0889-8561, ISBN-13: 978-0-323-68239-8

Editor: Jessica McCool

Developmental Editor: Kristen Helm

© **2019 Elsevier Inc. All rights reserved.**

This periodical and the individual contributions contained in it are protected under copyright by Elsevier, and the following terms and conditions apply to their use:

Photocopying

Single photocopies of single articles may be made for personal use as allowed by national copyright laws. Permission of the Publisher and payment of a fee is required for all other photocopying, including multiple or systematic copying, copying for advertising or promotional purposes, resale, and all forms of document delivery. Special rates are available for educational institutions that wish to make photocopies for non-profit educational classroom use. For information on how to seek permission visit www.elsevier.com/permissions or call: (+44) 1865 843830 (UK)/(+1) 215 239 3804 (USA).

Derivative Works

Subscribers may reproduce tables of contents or prepare lists of articles including abstracts for internal circulation within their institutions. Permission of the Publisher is required for resale or distribution outside the institution. Permission of the Publisher is required for all other derivative works, including compilations and translations (please consult www.elsevier.com/permissions).

Electronic Storage or Usage

Permission of the Publisher is required to store or use electronically any material contained in this periodical, including any article or part of an article (please consult www.elsevier.com/permissions). Except as outlined above, no part of this publication may be reproduced, stored in a retrieval system or transmitted in any form or by any means, electronic, mechanical, photocopying, recording or otherwise, without prior written permission of the Publisher.

Notice

No responsibility is assumed by the Publisher for any injury and/or damage to persons or property as a matter of products liability, negligence or otherwise, or from any use or operation of any methods, products, instructions or ideas contained in the material herein. Because of rapid advances in the medical sciences, in particular, independent verification of diagnoses and drug dosages should be made.

Although all advertising material is expected to conform to ethical (medical) standards, inclusion in this publication does not constitute a guarantee or endorsement of the quality or value of such product or of the claims made of it by its manufacturer.

Immunology and Allergy Clinics of North America (ISSN 0889–8561) is published quarterly by Elsevier Inc., 360 Park Avenue South, New York, NY 10010-1710. Months of issue are February, May, August, and November. Periodicals postage paid at New York, NY and additional mailing offices. Subscription prices are $341.00 per year for US individuals, $593.00 per year for US institutions, $100.00 per year for US students and residents, $423.00 per year for Canadian individuals, $220.00 per year for Canadian students, $753.00 per year for Canadian institutions, $447.00 per year for international individuals, $753.00 per year for international institutions, $220.00 per year for international students. To receive student/resident rate, orders must be accompanied by name of affiliated institution, date of term, and the *signature* of program/residency coordinator on institution letterhead. Orders will be billed at individual rate until proof of status is received. Foreign air speed delivery is included in all *Clinics* subscription prices. All prices are subject to change without notice. **POSTMASTER**: Send address changes to *Immunology and Allergy Clinics of North America,* Elsevier Health Sciences Division, Subscription Customer Service, 3251 Riverport Lane, Maryland Heights, MO 63043. **Customer Service: 1-800-654-2452 (U.S. and Canada); 314-447-8871 (outside U.S. and Canada). Fax: 314-447-8029. E-mail: journalscustomerservice-usa@elsevier.com (for print support); journalsonlinesupport-usa@elsevier.com (for online support).**

Reprints. For copies of 100 or more, of articles in this publication, please contact the Commercial Reprints Department, Elsevier Inc., 360 Park Avenue South, New York, New York 10010-1710. Tel. 212-633-3874, Fax: 212-633-3820, E-mail: reprints@elsevier.com.

Immunology and Allergy Clinics of North America is covered in MEDLINE/PubMed (Index Medicus), Current Contents/Life Sciences, Science Citation Index, ISI/BIOMED, Chemical Abstracts, and EMBASE/Excerpta Medica.

Printed in the United States of America.

Contributors

CONSULTING EDITOR

STEPHEN A. TILLES, MD
Senior Director, Aimmune Therapeutics, Clinical Professor of Medicine, University of Washington, Seattle, Washington, USA

EDITOR

MITCHELL H. GRAYSON, MD
Grant Morrow, III, MD, Endowed Chair in Pediatric Research, Professor and Chief, Division of Allergy and Immunology, Department of Pediatrics, The Ohio State University College of Medicine, Center for Translational and Clinical Research, The Research Institute at Nationwide Children's Hospital, Columbus, Ohio, USA

AUTHORS

LARRY BORISH, MD
Departments of Medicine and Microbiology, Carter Immunology Center, University of Virginia Health System, Charlottesville, Virginia, USA

LUCIANA SANTOS CARDOSO, PhD
Departamento de Análises Clínicas e Toxicológicas, Faculdade de Farmácia, Universidade Federal da Bahia, Salvador, Bahia, Brazil

ANDREA M. COVERSTONE, MD
Division of Allergy, Immunology and Pulmonary Medicine, Department of Pediatrics, Washington University School of Medicine, St Louis, Missouri, USA

ÁLVARO A. CRUZ, MD
ProAR - Universidade Federal da Bahia, Salvador, Bahia, Brazil

MAULI DESAI, MD
Associate Professor of Medicine, Division of Allergy and Clinical Immunology, Icahn School of Medicine at Mount Sinai, New York, New York, USA

ALEJANDRO DIAZ, MD
Center for Vaccines and Immunity, The Research Institute at Nationwide Children's Hospital, The Ohio State College of Medicine, Division of Infectious Diseases, Department of Pediatrics, Nationwide Children's Hospital, Columbus, Ohio, USA

JAMILLE SOUZA FERNANDES, PhD
Centro de Ciências Biológicas e da Saúde, Universidade Federal do Oeste da Bahia, Barreiras, Bahia, Brazil; ProAR - Universidade Federal da Bahia, Salvador, Bahia, Brazil

MITCHELL H. GRAYSON, MD
Grant Morrow, III, MD, Endowed Chair in Pediatric Research, Professor and Chief, Division of Allergy and Immunology, Department of Pediatrics, The Ohio State University College of Medicine, Center for Translational and Clinical Research, The Research Institute at Nationwide Children's Hospital, Columbus, Ohio, USA

MINGYUAN HAN, PhD
Postdoctoral Fellow, Department of Pediatrics and Communicable Diseases, University of Michigan Medical School, Ann Arbor, Michigan, USA

SANTTU HEINONEN, MD, PhD
New Children's Hospital, Pediatric Research Center, University of Helsinki, Helsinki University Hospital, Helsinki, Finland

MARC B. HERSHENSON, MD
Professor, Department of Pediatrics and Communicable Diseases, Department of Molecular and Integrative Physiology, University of Michigan Medical School, Ann Arbor, Michigan, USA

MICHAEL INSEL, MD
Fellow, Division of Pulmonary, Critical Care, Allergy, and Sleep Medicine, Department of Medicine, The University of Arizona Health Sciences, University of Arizona College of Medicine – Tucson, Tucson, Arizona, USA

JOSHUA L. KENNEDY, MD
Departments of Pediatrics and Internal Medicine, Arkansas Children's Research Institute, University of Arkansas for Medical Sciences, Little Rock, Arkansas, USA

MONICA KRAFT, MD
Chair, Department of Medicine, Asthma and Airway Disease Research Center, The University of Arizona Health Sciences, University of Arizona College of Medicine – Tucson, Tucson, Arizona, USA

JOAO PEDRO LOPES, MD
Clinical Fellow, Division of Allergy and Clinical Immunology, Icahn School of Medicine at Mount Sinai, New York, New York, USA

NICHOLAS W. LUKACS, PhD
Godfrey Dorr Stobbe Professor of Pathology, Assistant Dean for Faculty Affairs, Scientific Director, Mary H. Weiser Food Allergy Center, University of Michigan Medical School, Ann Arbor, Michigan, USA

ASUNCION MEJIAS, MD, PhD
Center for Vaccines and Immunity, The Research Institute at Nationwide Children's Hospital, Division of Infectious Diseases, Department of Pediatrics, Nationwide Children's Hospital, The Ohio State College of Medicine, Columbus, Ohio, USA; Department of Pharmacology and Pediatrics, Malaga Medical School, Malaga University (UMA), Spain

MARK E. PEEPLES, PhD
Principal Investigator, Center for Vaccines and Immunity, The Research Institute at Nationwide Children's Hospital, Professor, Department of Pediatrics, The Ohio State University College of Medicine, Columbus, Ohio, USA

SARAH PHAM, MD
Department of Pediatrics, University of Arkansas for Medical Sciences, Little Rock, Arkansas, USA

PAULO M. PITREZ, MD
Hospital Moinhos de Vento, Porto Alegre, Rio Grande do Sul, Brazil

CATHERINE PTASCHINSKI, PhD
Research Investigator, Department of Pathology, University of Michigan Medical School, Ann Arbor, Michigan, USA

CHARU RAJPUT, PhD
Postdoctoral Fellow, Department of Pediatrics and Communicable Diseases, University of Michigan Medical School, Ann Arbor, Michigan, USA

OCTAVIO RAMILO, MD
Center for Vaccines and Immunity, The Research Institute at Nationwide Children's Hospital, Division of Infectious Diseases, Department of Pediatrics, Nationwide Children's Hospital, The Ohio State College of Medicine, Columbus, Ohio, USA

JENNY RESILIAC, BA
Biomedical Sciences Graduate Program, Center for Translational and Clinical Research, The Research Institute at Nationwide Children's Hospital, Division of Allergy and Immunology, Department of Pediatrics, The Ohio State University College of Medicine, Columbus, Ohio, USA

ROSA RODRIGUEZ-FERNANDEZ, MD, PhD
Department of Pediatrics, Instituto de Investigación Sanitaria Gregorio Marañón (IISGM), Hospital Materno-Infantil Gregorio Marañón, Section of General Pediatrics, Hospital Gregorio Marañón, Madrid, Spain

SILVIA OLIVA RODRIGUEZ-PASTOR, MD
Division of Pediatric Emergency Medicine and Critical Care, Hospital Regional Universitario de Malaga, Malaga, Spain; Departamento de Farmacologia y Pediatria, Facultad de Medicina de Malaga, Universidad de Malaga, Spain

HOMERO SAN-JUAN-VERGARA, MD, PhD
Professor, Division of Health Sciences, Fundación Universidad del Norte, Universidad del Norte, Barranquilla, Colombia

ANNA G. STAUDACHER, MS
Division of Allergy and Immunology, Department of Medicine, Northwestern University Feinberg School of Medicine, Chicago, Illinois, USA

WHITNEY W. STEVENS, MD, PhD
Assistant Professor of Medicine, Division of Allergy and Immunology, Department of Medicine, Northwestern University Feinberg School of Medicine, Chicago, Illinois, USA

KAHARU SUMINO, MD, MPH
Division of Pulmonary and Critical Care Medicine, Department of Medicine, Washington University School of Medicine, St Louis, Missouri, USA

LEYAO WANG, PhD, MPH
Division of Pulmonary and Critical Care Medicine, Department of Medicine, Washington University School of Medicine, St Louis, Missouri, USA

Contents

Asthma and allergic diseases have become more prevalent, although the reasons for this increase in disease burden are not known. Understanding why these diseases have become more common requires knowledge of the disease pathogenesis. Multiple studies have identified respiratory viral infections and atypical bacteria as potential etiologic agents underlying the development of asthma (and possibly allergies). This review discusses the epidemiology and potential mechanistic studies that provide links between these infectious agents and the development (and exacerbation) of asthma. These studies provide insight into the increase in disease prevalence and have identified potential targets for future therapeutic intervention.

The infant's developing immune response is central to establishing a balanced system that reacts appropriately to infectious stimuli, but does not induce altered disease states with potential long-term sequelae. Respiratory syncytial virus may alter the immune system, affecting future responses. Early infection may have direct effects on the lung itself. Other early life processes contribute to the development of immune responses including assembly of the microbiome, which seems to have a particularly important role for establishing the immune environment. This review covers studies that have set up important paradigms and discusses recent data that direct research toward informative hypotheses.

Severe lower respiratory tract infection in infants and young children is most frequently caused by respiratory syncytial virus (RSV). RSV infects the smallest airways, making breathing difficult and in some infants requiring medical support. Severity is affected by viral dose, infant age, virus genotype, and effectiveness of the innate/adaptive immune responses. Severe disease correlates with later wheezing and asthma in some children. The adaptive immune response is protective but wanes after each infection, likely due to the ability of the RSV NS1/NS2 proteins to inhibit the innate immune response. Several vaccine approaches and candidates are currently in clinical trials.

of neonates promote immune maturation and protect against asthma pathogenesis. Later bacterial infections and perturbations to the microbiome can contribute to asthma pathogenesis, persistence, and severity.

Respiratory viruses other than rhinovirus or respiratory syncytial virus, including human metapneumovirus, influenza virus, and human bocavirus, are important pathogens in acute wheezing illness and asthma exacerbations in young children. Whether infection with these viruses in early life is associated with recurrent wheezing and/or asthma is not fully investigated, although there are data to suggest children with human metapneumovirus lower respiratory tract infection may have a higher likelihood of subsequent and recurrent wheezing several years after initial infection.

There is an important link between the upper and lower respiratory tracts whereby inflammation in one environment can influence the other. In acute rhinosinusitis, pathogen exposures are the primary driver for inflammation in the nose, which can exacerbate asthma. In chronic rhinosinusitis, a disease clinically associated with asthma, the inflammation observed is likely from a combination of an impaired epithelial barrier, dysregulated immune response, and potentially infection (or colonization) by specific pathogens. This review explores the associations between rhinosinusitis and asthma, with particular emphasis placed on the role of infections and inflammation.

Helminth infections may inhibit the development of allergic diseases, including asthma. On the other hand, some helminth species may induce or worsen symptoms of asthma. This article discusses the impact of helminth infections on asthma as well as the potencial of helminth-derived molecules with regulatory characteristics in the prevention or treatment of this disease. The ability to induce regulation has been observed in animal models of asthma or cells of asthmatic individuals in vitro. Potential future clinical applications of helminth antigens or infection for prevention of asthma merit further translational research.

Monoclonal antibodies block specific inflammatory pathways involved in the pathogenesis of asthma. These pathways, such as immunoglobulin E and interleukin 5 pathways, are important in host defense against pathogens, in particular against parasites. Despite theoretic concerns about infection risk, biologics seem to have a favorable safety profile. Data from large clinical trials and postmarketing surveillance for these drugs have not shown increases in severe infections, including those from parasitic organisms. This may be due to redundancy of effector cells within the immune system. Certain drugs have special considerations and precautions; therefore, the prescribing physician should be familiar with product recommendations and warnings. Given the short-term nature of clinical trials (most are under 52 weeks) and the emergence of many new biologics on the market, continued pharmacovigilance is vital to assess long-term safety.

IMMUNOLOGY AND ALLERGY CLINICS OF NORTH AMERICA

SERIES OF RELATED INTEREST

Infectious Disease Clinics of North America
Available at: https://www.id.theclinics.com/

THE CLINICS ARE AVAILABLE ONLINE!
Access your subscription at:
www.theclinics.com

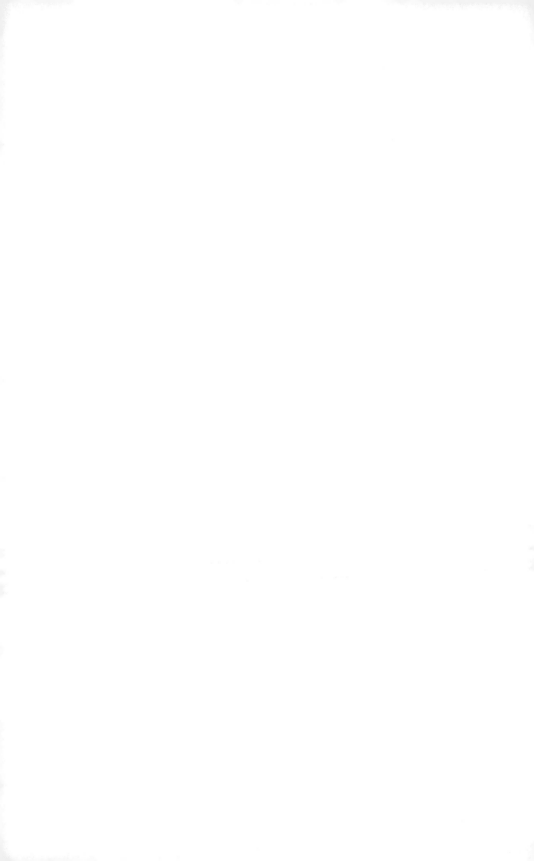

Foreword

Microbes, Infections, and Their Relationship to Asthma

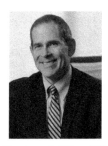

Stephen A. Tilles, MD
Consulting Editor

Examining the impact of bacteria, viruses, fungi, and parasites on human disease has been a complicated undertaking that began centuries ago and has led to profound effects on human history, including the development of interventions such as sanitation technologies, antibiotics, and vaccinations. In recent decades, we have also begun to appreciate the potential detrimental effects of altering natural patterns of microbial species that coexist with us, including the importance of changes in the early-life microbiome on the development of asthma and other allergic diseases.

Although asthma is typically thought of as an allergic disease, the roles of infections are arguably as complex and fundamental to asthma pathogenesis as allergens. Textbook chapters and patient education materials routinely list "respiratory infections" as environmental factors that both catalyze the development of asthma in genetically predisposed individuals and serve as classic exacerbation triggers for preexisting asthma. The best-understood microbes serving these roles are respiratory syncytial virus and rhinovirus, although our understanding of the exact mechanisms through which these viruses result in asthma flares is incomplete. For example, rhinovirus is well known to thrive at the relatively cool temperature of the upper airway, yet it somehow exerts a profound acute exacerbating effect on asthma, and this effect is enhanced during infections occurring in the presence of an allergen cofactor, such as springtime pollen. This is a fascinating story, but there is still disagreement whether rhinoviruses cause exacerbations directly within the lung itself or via circulating immunologic mediators.

Dr Tilles' consultant work for this issue of *Immunology and Allergy Clinics of North America* was completed before he became an employee of Aimmune Therapeutics.

This issue of *Immunology and Allergy Clinics of North America* focuses on the effects of viruses and other microbes on asthma. Editor Mitchell Grayson has assembled an impressive group of authors to contribute to this collection of articles, which separately are interesting focused reviews and together comprise a comprehensive overview of the subject. Topics range from the epidemiology of infections in asthma, to the importance of early-life viral infections, to the role of bacterial infections. There are also articles reviewing the often-protective role of helminth infection, and the impact of asthma biologic therapies on the risk of infections. I highly recommend this issue as a valuable reference for all health care providers who manage asthma patients as well as clinical and translational researchers.

Stephen A. Tilles, MD
Medical Affairs
Aimmune Therapeutics
8000 Marina Boulevard #200
Brisbane, CA 94005, USA

University of Washington
Seattle, WA 98105, USA

E-mail address:
stilles@aimmune.com

Preface

The Complicated Dance of Infections and Asthma

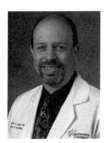

Mitchell H. Grayson, MD
Editor

The interaction between asthma and infections is a complicated one, and that is the focus of this issue of the *Immunology and Allergy Clinics of North America*. Infections, both viral and bacterial, have been associated with development and exacerbation of asthma, while parasitic infections may actually help protect against asthma. Furthermore, as our drug armamentarium begins to focus on biologics, which can selectively impair components of the immune response, there is concern that treated patients with asthma will be at risk of developing opportunistic infections.

To fully put the role of infections and asthma into context, this issue starts with an overview of the epidemiology of infections and asthma. This is followed by a discussion of the virus most often associated with development of asthma, respiratory syncytial virus (RSV), and the mechanisms that have been shown to link RSV infection to the development of asthma. Recent research on RSV has identified characteristics of the virus that may play a role in the development of asthma, and 1 article examines the role of RSV-specific characteristics in this process and the potential for an RSV vaccine. Another virus, human rhinovirus (RV), is the cause of the common cold and the virus most often associated with asthma exacerbations. In this issue, the role RV plays in this process is explored, from both an epidemiologic standpoint and the mechanistic components leading from RV infection to asthma exacerbation. With all of these viral insults, it is less the virus than the resulting immune response that drives development or exacerbation of disease. Studies are beginning to better elucidate the immune response to respiratory viruses, especially in infants, and this is discussed as well.

RSV and RV are not the only viruses associated with asthma exacerbations and development. We include a discussion of other viruses that appear to play an important role. In fact, bacteria have a significant impact on asthma development and exacerbation. The role of these bacteria is explored, both when the bacteria are a foreign invader (ie, an infection) or when they are an important friend (ie, the microbiome). Infections

Immunol Allergy Clin N Am 39 (2019) xv–xvi
https://doi.org/10.1016/j.iac.2019.04.002
0889-8561/19/© 2019 Published by Elsevier Inc.

outside the lung can also exacerbate asthma, and the emerging role of sinus infections as a cause of asthma exacerbations is explored, focusing on the potential mechanisms linking these 2 diseases.

We include the potential role of helminths, although not often considered in a discussion of asthma. Recent work suggests helminths may protect against asthma exacerbations, and this could be exploited for therapeutic benefit. Finally, with the advent of biologic therapies to treat asthma, the potential for infectious complications in patients with asthma treated with these medications is explored.

This truly is a whirlwind tour of the state-of-the-art of infections and asthma, and I hope you find it exciting and thought provoking. I would be amiss if I did not thank all of the world-class contributors who have made this such an important and interesting issue. I have learned greatly by editing this issue and hope you do, too. In addition, I wish to thank the staff at *Immunology and Allergy Clinics of North America*, and especially Kristen Helm, for keeping everyone focused and on task, and Dr Stephen Tilles, for the opportunity to explore this topic. Great strides have been made in understanding the relationship between infectious agents and asthma, but as discussed through the articles in this issue, much is still to be learned.

Mitchell H. Grayson, MD
Division of Allergy and Immunology
Department of Pediatrics
Nationwide Children's Hospital
The Ohio State University College of Medicine
700 Children's Drive
Columbus, OH 43205, USA

E-mail addresses:
wheeze@allergist.com; Mitchell.Grayson@Nationwidechildrens.org

Epidemiology of Infections and Development of Asthma

Jenny Resiliac, BA[a,b,c], Mitchell H. Grayson, MD[a,b,c],*

KEYWORDS

- Asthma • Allergy • Respiratory virus • Atypical bacteria • Epidemiology

KEY POINTS

- Respiratory RNA viral infections have been correlated with the development and exacerbation of asthma (and possibly allergies).
- Atypical bacteria and some typical bacteria have also been associated with asthma development.
- The mechanisms linking these organisms to development and exacerbation of asthma are areas actively being explored.

INTRODUCTION

Asthma is a common chronic condition affecting both children and adults and is characterized by chronic airway inflammation leading to bronchial hyperresponsiveness and mucous hypersecretion. Asthma can be triggered by a variety of stimuli, leading to recurrent and reversible episodes of wheezing, shortness of breath, chest tightness, and coughing.[1] Asthma prevalence has increased dramatically both in the United States and worldwide. Recent statistics from the National Health Interview Surveys and the US Centers for Disease Control and Prevention estimated that 26.5 million

Disclosures: J. Resiliac has no disclosures; M.H. Grayson is the editor of this edition of *Immunology and Allergy Clinics*, has been on the advisory board for AstraZeneca, has received research funds from the National Institutes of Health and the Research Institute at Nationwide Children's Hospital, is an Associate Editor for the *Annals of Allergy, Asthma, and Immunology*, and is on the board of directors of the American Board of Allergy and Immunology, the Asthma and Allergy Foundation of America, and the American Academy of Allergy, Asthma, and Immunology.
Funded by: NIH Grant number(s): HL087778, NIHMS-ID: 1523912.
[a] Center for Translational and Clinical Research, The Research Institute at Nationwide Children's Hospital, 700 Children's Drive, Columbus, OH 43205, USA; [b] Biomedical Sciences Graduate Program, The Ohio State University College of Medicine, Columbus, OH, USA; [c] Division of Allergy and Immunology, Department of Pediatrics, The Ohio State University College of Medicine, Columbus, OH, USA
* Corresponding author. Division of Allergy and Immunology, Nationwide Children's Hospital, 700 Children's Drive, Columbus, OH 43205.
E-mail address: wheeze@allergist.com

Immunol Allergy Clin N Am 39 (2019) 297–307
https://doi.org/10.1016/j.iac.2019.03.001
0889-8561/19/© 2019 Elsevier Inc. All rights reserved.

people in the United States, including 6.1 million children, have asthma.[2] Globally, about 235 million people suffer from asthma.[3] Implicated in the development of asthma are respiratory viral infections and infections with atypical bacteria (such as mycoplasma and/or chlamydia). Infectious agents have not only been associated with the inception of disease in asthma, they have also been involved in its exacerbations. In fact, in 2015 more than 11.5 million people with asthma, including nearly 3 million children, had 1 or more exacerbations of their asthma.[4] The burden of asthma is significant, both in terms of financial expenses and lost productivity, and in many situations it is an infectious agent that initiates an asthma exacerbation. This review discusses the epidemiology of respiratory infections (**Fig. 1**) in the development of asthma, as well as potential mechanisms that may translate these respiratory infections into asthma.

EPIDEMIOLOGY OF INFECTIONS AND ASTHMA

The role of early life infections in the development of asthma results from complex interactions between pathogens, genetics, and environmental factors such as tobacco smoke. Acute respiratory infections are common in asthmatic patients. Although controversial, some investigators believe there may be an increased risk of infection among atopic patients caused by opportunistic infections, especially in patients with severe atopic diseases.[5] For instance, viral or bacterial infections were observed in 70% of adult inpatients with an asthma exacerbation[6] and clinical studies report that

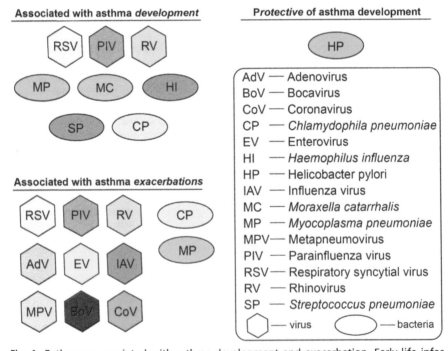

Fig. 1. Pathogens associated with asthma development and exacerbation. Early life infections play a role in the development of asthma and disease exacerbation. This figure lists the pathogens that have been associated with asthma development (*upper left*) and asthma exacerbations (*bottom left*). *Helicobacter pylori* has been shown to be protective of asthma development (*upper right*). Abbreviations are explained in the box; viruses are shown in hexagrams, and bacteria are in ovals. See text for more details.

asthma onset after an acute respiratory illness is exceedingly common (up to 45% of adult-onset asthma cases).[7] Of course, this finding just supports the idea that respiratory infections can exacerbate asthma, but does not prove that patients with asthma are more likely to have a respiratory infection. A study comparing more than 11,000 individuals reported an increased risk of developing asthma in individuals who had any infection independent of their smoking history.[8] Individuals with early asthma who never smoked had significantly increased risk of any infection (hazard ratio [HR], 1.65; 95% confidence interval [CI], 1.40–1.94), pneumonia (HR, 2.44; 95% CI, 1.92–3.11) or any nonrespiratory tract infection (HR, 1.36; 95% CI, 1.11–1.67); results were similar in smokers with early asthma. The researchers also found that asthma history was not limited to early disease because individuals who never smoked but had any history of asthma during their lifetime also had significantly increased risk of infection (HR, 1.44; 95% CI, 1.24–1.66) and pneumonia (HR, 1.99; 95% CI, 1.62–2.44).[8] However, there remains the issue of bias—those with asthma are more likely to have clinically significant infections. Finally, not surprisingly, early infections but not smoking history were the best indicators for the development of asthma.

VIRAL INFECTIONS AND DEVELOPMENT OF ASTHMA

As mentioned, evidence supports the role of early life viral infections in the development of asthma. Viral infections are common during early childhood development. Infant respiratory viral infection and childhood asthma are the most common acute and chronic diseases of childhood, respectively.[9] So, it is not surprising that these 2 illnesses overlap. Bronchiolitis and early wheezing are frequently seen in children, usually as a result of a viral infection (regardless of the presence of asthma). Respiratory viruses often are detected in first-time wheezing children and may associate with the development of atopic disease.[10] Studies have shown that one-third of all children suffer from infection-induced wheezing during the first 3 years of life.[11,12] Up to one-half of all children have acute wheezing at least once before school age, and among these children, 30% to 40% develop recurrent wheezing.[11] Moreover, viral respiratory infections have been implicated in up to 80% of wheezing episodes and asthma exacerbations.[13] These studies demonstrate the relationship of viral infections and development or wheezing and/or exacerbation of asthma.

Respiratory syncytial virus (RSV), rhinovirus (RV), and parainfluenza viruses (parainfluenza viruses 1 and 2) are most commonly detected in asthma exacerbations in children, but they have been associated as well in the development of the disease—especially with severe infections by these viruses early in life.[14–17] Wheezing illnesses in infancy and early childhood caused by viral infection of RV, RSV, and parainfluenza strongly correlate with asthma development later in life.[18–20] Although RSV and RV seem to be the viruses most associated with asthma development, a larger group of pathogens have been identified in asthma exacerbations (see **Fig. 1**). Within the range of these respiratory viral pathogens, the most common viruses identified during an asthma exacerbation are RV (44%–88%), RSV (2%–20%), and parainfluenza virus (2%–11%).[21] Other viruses associated with asthma exacerbations (usually <5% of the time) include adenovirus, enterovirus (EV; non-RV), influenza, metapneumovirus, bocavirus, and coronovirus.[22,23] It is also important to note that around 10% of these cases have a coinfection with more than 1 virus—usually with RV being the other virus identified.[24]

RESPIRATORY SYNCYTIAL VIRUS AND THE DEVELOPMENT OF ASTHMA

The initial studies linking respiratory viral infections with development of asthma focused on RSV, which is one of the most common infections in children and infants.

RSV is also known as one of the leading causes of severe respiratory infection in infants and several studies have strongly suggested a causal role for RSV in the development of asthma and allergen sensitization.[24–27] A cohort study by El Saleeby and colleagues[28] found that high levels of RSV titer were associated with more severe respiratory viral disease outcomes. In this study, previously healthy RSV-infected children under 2 years old who had significantly higher viral titers had increased requirements for intensive medical care and were more prone to respiratory failure when compared with those with lower titers.[28] Asthma outcomes were similarly affected as demonstrated by a multicenter cohort study in the United States and Finland conducted by Hasegawa and colleagues,[29] determining the relationship between viral load in RSV-infected children and clinical symptoms of asthma. Out of the 2612 children in the study, 67% developed RSV bronchiolitis, but most interestingly, children with higher RSV titers had a higher risk for severe bronchiolitis.[29] Taken together, these studies demonstrate the relevance of severe RSV infections in the development of asthma and asthma symptoms.

ENTEROVIRUSES AND ASTHMA

EV are RNA viruses of the family *Picornaviridae*, of which the most common is RV, which has been associated with asthma development and exacerbation.[30] The Childhood Origins of ASThma (COAST) cohort study followed children from birth and identified RV as the viral etiology of 90% of wheezing illnesses by age 3 years; RV was identified as the major risk factor for asthma at 6 years of age.[21] Although RV is associated with asthma development, the COAST investigators used mathematical modeling to demonstrate that RV infection likely followed the development of atopy. This finding raises a question as to whether respiratory RV infections drive development of asthma, or simply uncover an existing predisposition for the disease.

RV can be divided into 3 clades, RV-A, RV-B, and RV-C. Of these 3, RV-C has been found to most strongly correlate with severity of asthma exacerbations.[23] A recent study from China further verified that RV-C is associated most often with both inpatient and outpatient asthma exacerbations, but also demonstrated that high titer of RV-A also could lead to significant exacerbation of disease.[24] Clearly, RV is a major component of asthma disease burden, even if it is not a causative of disease development.

In addition to RV, other EV have been identified in patients undergoing an asthma exacerbation, and these viruses may play a role in the inception of asthma. Many studies have reported an association with an increased incidence of EV infections and asthma development.[31–34] One study retrospectively compared patients over a decade (January 2000 to December 2011) and examined the relationship between EV infection and asthma. The incidence of asthma was 1.48-fold higher in patients (≤5 years old) who had an EV infection compared with those who did not.[35] Although the results were intriguing, it is important to note that this was a retrospective study depending on claims data.

INFLUENZA AND ASTHMA

Influenza circulates both as a seasonal infection and occasional pandemic. The seasonal variety clearly causes asthma exacerbations, but seems to be a minor contributor to the overall burden of asthma disease development. During the 2009 influenza pandemic (pH1N1), asthma was the most common comorbidity among patients, accounting for 22% to 29% of all hospitalized patients with influenza.[36–39] Children with asthma accounted for 44% of hospitalized children with influenza, although the major differences between the pandemic influenza and seasonal influenza was that pH1N1 was associated with higher incidence of pneumonia (46% vs 40%, pH1N1 vs seasonal, respectively; P = .04) and a greater need for intensive care (22% vs 16%; P = .01).[40] Another study analyzed data from 12 different Canadian pediatrics hospitals during the pH1N1 pandemic and compared them with data from children hospitalized with seasonal influenza A. The results from that study revealed that preexisting asthma was overrepresented in pH1N1 infected relative to seasonal influenza A infections.[41] Further, pH1N1 seemed to cause more disease in older children, with the median age for these pH1N1 patients being 4.8 years old, whereas the median age for seasonal influenza A patients was 1.7 years.[41] Data from 272 patients hospitalized for at least 24 hours with an influenza-like illness and a positive H1N1 polymerase chain reaction test demonstrated that 73% of the patients had at least 1 underlying medical condition; these conditions included asthma, diabetes, pregnancy, and other heart, lung, and neurologic diseases.[36] Although asthma was overrepresented in patients hospitalized with pH1N1, at least 1 study found that having asthma led to a more rapid recovery from the viral infection.[42] Supporting the idea that asthma might have a protective advantage in the recovery from pH1N1, a retrospective chart review of 2 case series found that those with asthma who were hospitalized with pH1N1 were less likely to have pneumonia, need mechanical ventilation, or die compared with those admitted without asthma.[42] So, although influenza may be associated with asthma exacerbations, it also seems that asthma may protect against pandemic influenza mediated morbidity and mortality.

The mechanisms linking respiratory viral infections to development of asthma and its exacerbation are actively being studied. Some links relate to the role of innate lymphoid cells (ILCs), translating RSV infection into atopic disease. ILCs can be classified based on their transcriptional regulation and cytokine production into ILC1, ILC2, and ILC3 cells, which largely emulate the adaptive CD4$^+$ T helper 1 (Th1), Th2, and Th17 cells, respectively. ILC2s produce high levels of IL-13 and IL-5, 2 cytokines known to play important roles in asthma. IL-5 is a required cytokine for eosinophil development, and several new asthma treatments have been developed to block its effects.[43] IL-13 has been implicated in IgE synthesis, mucus hypersecretion, airway hyperresponsiveness, and fibrosis.[44] In a murine model, RSV induced robust IL-13 production from ILC2 during the early phase of the infection.[45] This increased production of IL-13 was found to depend on thymic stromal lymphopoietin signaling. Neutralizing thymic stromal lymphopoietin resulted in significant reduction of IL-13 and the postviral airway disease.[45]

We have used the murine parainfluenza virus, Sendai virus (SeV), to explore the translation of a respiratory viral infection into asthma. Mice infected with SeV develop postviral airway hyperreactivity and mucous cell metaplasia after clearance of the virus. The mechanistic pathway depends on the initial recruitment of a subset of CD49d expressing neutrophils, which require cysteinyl leukotrienes for their survival. These neutrophils induce expression of the high-affinity receptor for IgE, FcεRI, on lung conventional dendritic cells (DC). At the same time the mouse makes IgE against SeV, and this leads to cross-linking of FcεRI on the DC. This crosslinking of DC FcεRI induces the production of CCL28, a chemokine that recruits IL-13–producing lymphocytes to the lung. The IL-13 then drives subsequent development of postviral airway disease.[46] Interestingly, exposure to a nonviral antigen during the antiviral immune response is sufficient to drive allergic disease against the nonviral antigen. Thus, this model translates a respiratory viral infection into atopy and asthma. Importantly, components of this pathway are present in the human. We demonstrated CD49d expressing neutrophils in the nasal lavage of humans and expression of the cysteinyl leukotriene receptor on these cells.[47] Human conventional DC express FcεRI, and the level of expression is increased during a respiratory viral infection.[48] Cross-linking DC FcεRI leads to release of CCL28, and humans make IgE against viruses, such as RSV and RV.[49–54] Whether this pathway does indeed translate a respiratory viral infection to asthma in human infants remains to be fully determined.

ATYPICAL BACTERIAL INFECTION AND THE DEVELOPMENT OF ASTHMA

Infections with atypical bacteria also seem to play a role in the induction and exacerbation of asthma in both children and adults. Several studies suggest that atypical respiratory pathogens such as *Chlamydophila pneumoniae* (CP) and *Mycoplasma pneumoniae* (MP) and fungi like *Aspergillosis* may contribute to the pathogenesis of asthma.[55–59] Chronic CP infections are more frequent in asthmatic patients and have been associated with poor asthma control.[60,61] Von and colleagues[62] investigated the relationship between severity of asthma, CP titers, and antibodies specific for CP's heat shock protein (chsp60), and their association with asthma. Patients (n = 116) were categorized into 3 groups based on the severity of their asthma (mild, moderate, or severe). Although antibodies against chsp60 were elevated in the asthmatic group compared with the controls, the difference did not reach statistical significance. However, severe and moderate asthma were significantly associated with the presence of elevated anti-chsp60 IgA, suggesting chronic infection in these patients with more severe asthma.[62] An additional study reported that IgE against CP strongly and positively associated with asthma severity, suggesting a role of anti-CP IgE (and by extension, CP) in the pathogenesis of asthma.[63] Although MP's role in asthma has been less intensively investigated than CP, MP has been associated with recurrent wheeze and may be present as a coinfection with respiratory viruses. Children with asthma were more likely to have MP-specific IgM than those without asthma (39% vs 0%),[64] suggesting an increased exposure and colonization of MP in those with asthma.

In addition to CP and MP, emerging data suggest species of the *Streptococcus*, *Moraxella*, and *Haemophilus* genera also associate with respiratory illnesses and asthma development.[65,66] Hypopharyngeal colonization with *S pneumoniae*, *Helicobacter influenza*, or *M catarrhalis* in neonates was reported to increase the risk for recurrent wheeze and asthma early in life.[67] In neonates, colonization with *H influenza* or *M catarrhalis* (or both) significantly associated with persistent wheeze (HR, 2.40; 95% CI, 1.45–3.99), acute severe exacerbation of wheeze (HR, 2.99; 95% CI, 1.66–5.39), and hospitalization for wheeze (HR, 3.85; 95% CI, 1.90–7.79).[67] In fact, children colonized by these bacteria as neonates had a higher prevalence of asthma by 5 years of age, as well as increased beta-agonist reversibility compared with those children not colonized as neonates with these organisms. Other bacteria such as *Helicobacter pylori* and *Bordetella pertussis* have been associated with asthma, as well. In subjects under 40 years of age, *H pylori* infection (as documented by IgG against *H pylori* in the peripheral blood) seems to protect against asthma (odds ratio [OR], 0.503), but not other allergic diseases.[68] *B pertussis* has not been associated with the development of asthma, but may infect asthma patients more frequently. After a pertussis outbreak in California and Minnesota, Capili and colleagues[69] conducted a population-based, case-control study to determine the prevalence of pertussis and its association with asthma. They reported an increased risk of *B pertussis* infection among subjects with asthma (adjusted OR for *B pertussis* infection with preexisting asthma, 1.73; 95% CI, 1.12–2.67; P = .013). Interestingly, the majority of this risk was attributable to children (OR, 1.92; 95% CI, 1.2–3.09; P = .007) but not adults (OR, 1.14; 95% CI,

0.37–3.55; P = .820). These authors calculated the population attributable risk of asthma for pertussis infection at 17%.[69] Thus, bacterial infections can have implications beyond just the development and/or exacerbation of asthma.

Similar to viral infections, the mechanisms by which atypical bacterial drive the inception of asthma are being studied. Early infection with CP or MP leads to a higher risk for asthma through induction of type 2 airway inflammation, mucus cell metaplasia, and airway hyperreactivity, all hallmarks of asthma. For instance, CP infection was shown to induce a Th2 immune response, as well as both airway eosinophilia and neutrophilia leading to permanent alteration of lung structure and function.[70] Using a mouse model, it was shown that infection with a chlamydia species (*C muridarum*) during allergen sensitization (using ovalbumin) led to a neutrophilic inflammatory response in the lung associated with a Th1/Th17 response, but an inhibited Th2 response.[71] This model is reminiscent of the human neutrophilic asthma phenotype. If CP and MP do cause asthma, then treatment with macrolide antibiotics (for which CP and MP are sensitive) should prevent or ameliorate asthma. In fact, treatment with a macrolide antibiotic in vitro did block CP-induced mucin production in cultured human airway cells.[72] A larger clinical study found that macrolide treatment decreased the severity of respiratory tract infections, but had no impact on the symptom scores or the use of albuterol.[73] Therefore, it remains unclear how important atypical bacterial infections are to the pathogenesis of asthma.

SUMMARY

This review has discussed the association between various respiratory pathogens and the development and exacerbation of asthma. Viral respiratory infections are common causes of acute illnesses in both adults and children, and are strongly associated with the inception and exacerbation of asthma. As discussed, several other pathogens, such as atypical bacteria like CP and MP, also have been linked to the onset and exacerbation of asthma. Some microorganisms (like *H pylori*) have a protective effect against the development of asthma. Further studies are required to better outline the complex interaction between human hosts and pathogens that lead to (or prevent) asthma development. These studies will require multidisciplinary approaches, including epidemiologic studies with longitudinal cohorts and mechanistic mouse models. These future investigations will increase our knowledge of the pathologic process during infections that lead to the development of asthma and will enable us to identify new therapeutic targets. These future interventions hopefully will decrease and perhaps eliminate the development and exacerbations of asthma.

REFERENCES

1. National Asthma Education and Prevention Program. National Asthma Education and Prevention Program. Expert panel report: guidelines for the diagnosis and management of asthma update on selected topics–2002. J Allergy Clin Immunol 2002;110(5 Suppl):S141–219.
2. United States Center for Disease Control and Prevention. Most recent asthma data. Available at: https://www.cdc.gov/asthma/most_recent_data.htm. Accessed October 15, 2018.
3. World Health Organization. Asthma. Available at: http://www.who.int/news-room/fact-sheets/detail/asthma. Accessed October 15, 2018.
4. United States Center for Disease Control and Prevention. 2015 National Health Interview Survey (NHIS) Data. Available at: https://www.cdc.gov/asthma/nhis/2015/table5-1.htm. Accessed October 15, 2018.

5. Juhn YJ. Risks for infection in patients with asthma (or other atopic conditions): is asthma more than a chronic airway disease? J Allergy Clin Immunol 2014;134(2): 247–57 [quiz: 258–9].

6. Iikura M, Hojo M, Koketsu R, et al. The importance of bacterial and viral infections associated with adult asthma exacerbations in clinical practice. PLoS One 2015; 10(4):e0123584.

7. Hahn DL. Infectious asthma: a reemerging clinical entity? J Fam Pract 1995; 41(2):153–7.

8. Helby J, Nordestgaard BG, Benfield T, et al. Asthma, other atopic conditions and risk of infections in 105 519 general population never and ever smokers. J Intern Med 2017;282(3):254–67.

9. Busse WW, Lemanske RF Jr, Gern JE. Role of viral respiratory infections in asthma and asthma exacerbations. Lancet 2010;376(9743):826–34.

10. Turunen R, Koistinen A, Vuorinen T, et al. The first wheezing episode: respiratory virus etiology, atopic characteristics, and illness severity. Pediatr Allergy Immunol 2014;25(8):796–803.

11. Taussig LM, Wright AL, Holberg CJ, et al. Tucson children's respiratory study: 1980 to present. J Allergy Clin Immunol 2003;111(4):661–75 [quiz: 676].

12. Piippo-Savolainen E, Korppi M. Long-term outcomes of early childhood wheezing. Curr Opin Allergy Clin Immunol 2009;9(3):190–6.

13. Carroll KN, Hartert TV. The impact of respiratory viral infection on wheezing illnesses and asthma exacerbations. Immunol Allergy Clin North Am 2008;28(3): 539–61, viii.

14. Wu P, Hartert TV. Evidence for a causal relationship between respiratory syncytial virus infection and asthma. Expert Rev Anti Infect Ther 2011;9(9):731–45.

15. Shay DK, Holman RC, Newman RD, et al. Bronchiolitis-associated hospitalizations among US children, 1980-1996. JAMA 1999;282(15):1440–6.

16. Wos M, Sanak M, Soja J, et al. The presence of rhinovirus in lower airways of patients with bronchial asthma. Am J Respir Crit Care Med 2008;177(10):1082–9.

17. Lee WM, Kiesner C, Pappas T, et al. A diverse group of previously unrecognized human rhinoviruses are common causes of respiratory illnesses in infants. PLoS One 2007;2(10):e966.

18. Blomqvist S, Roivainen M, Puhakka T, et al. Virological and serological analysis of rhinovirus infections during the first two years of life in a cohort of children. J Med Virol 2002;66(2):263–8.

19. Rossi GA, Colin AA. Infantile respiratory syncytial virus and human rhinovirus infections: respective role in inception and persistence of wheezing. Eur Respir J 2015;45(3):774–89.

20. Kneyber MCJ, Steyerberg EW, de Groot R, et al. Long-term effects of respiratory syncytial virus (RSV) bronchiolitis in infants and young children: a quantitative review. Acta Paediatr 2000;89(6):654–60.

21. Jackson DJ, Gangnon RE, Evans MD, et al. Wheezing rhinovirus illnesses in early life predict asthma development in high-risk children. Am J Respir Crit Care Med 2008;178(7):667–72.

22. Tregoning JS, Schwarze J. Respiratory viral infections in infants: causes, clinical symptoms, virology, and immunology. Clin Microbiol Rev 2010;23(1):74–98.

23. Bizzintino J, Lee WM, Laing IA, et al. Association between human rhinovirus C and severity of acute asthma in children. Eur Respir J 2011;37(5):1037–42.

24. Zheng SY, Wang LL, Ren L, et al. Epidemiological analysis and follow-up of human rhinovirus infection in children with asthma exacerbation. J Med Virol 2018;90(2):219–28.

25. Sigurs N, Bjarnason R, Sigurbergsson F, et al. Asthma and immunoglobulin E antibodies after respiratory syncytial virus bronchiolitis: a prospective cohort study with matched controls. Pediatrics 1995;95(4):500–5.
26. Sigurs N, Aljassim F, Kjellman B, et al. Asthma and allergy patterns over 18 years after severe RSV bronchiolitis in the first year of life. Thorax 2010;65(12):1045–52.
27. Welliver RC. RSV and chronic asthma. Lancet 1995;346(8978):789–90.
28. El Saleeby CM, Bush AJ, Harrison LM, et al. Respiratory syncytial virus load, viral dynamics, and disease severity in previously healthy naturally infected children. J Infect Dis 2011;204(7):996–1002.
29. Hasegawa K, Jartti T, Mansbach JM, et al. Respiratory syncytial virus genomic load and disease severity among children hospitalized with bronchiolitis: multicenter cohort studies in the United States and Finland. J Infect Dis 2015; 211(10):1550–9.
30. Lemanske RF Jr, Jackson DJ, Gangnon RE, et al. Rhinovirus illnesses during infancy predict subsequent childhood wheezing. J Allergy Clin Immunol 2005; 116(3):571–7.
31. Moss RB. Enterovirus 68 infection–association with asthma. J Allergy Clin Immunol Pract 2016;4(2):226–8.
32. Foster CB, Coelho R, Brown PM, et al. A comparison of hospitalized children with enterovirus D68 to those with rhinovirus. Pediatr Pulmonol 2017;52(6):827–32.
33. Moyer K, Wang H, Salamon D, et al. Enterovirus D68 in hospitalized children: sequence variation, viral loads and clinical outcomes. PLoS One 2016;11(11): e0167111.
34. Wang YC, Tsai CS, Yang YH, et al. Association between enterovirus infection and asthma in children: a 16-year nationwide population-based cohort study. Pediatr Infect Dis J 2018;37(9):844–9.
35. Yeh JJ, Lin CL, Hsu WH. Effect of enterovirus infections on asthma in young children: a national cohort study. Eur J Clin Invest 2017;47(12).
36. Jain S, Kamimoto L, Bramley AM, et al. Hospitalized patients with 2009 H1N1 influenza in the United States, April-June 2009. N Engl J Med 2009;361(20): 1935–44.
37. O'Riordan S, Barton M, Yau Y, et al. Risk factors and outcomes among children admitted to hospital with pandemic H1N1 influenza. CMAJ 2010;182(1):39–44.
38. Kloepfer KM, Olenec JP, Lee WM, et al. Increased H1N1 infection rate in children with asthma. Am J Respir Crit Care Med 2012;185(12):1275–9.
39. Myles P, Nguyen-Van-Tam JS, Semple MG, et al. Differences between asthmatics and nonasthmatics hospitalised with influenza A infection. Eur Respir J 2013; 41(4):824–31.
40. Dawood FS, Kamimoto L, D'Mello TA, et al. Children with asthma hospitalized with seasonal or pandemic influenza, 2003-2009. Pediatrics 2011;128(1):e27–32.
41. Tran D, Vaudry W, Moore DL, et al. Comparison of children hospitalized with seasonal versus pandemic influenza A, 2004-2009. Pediatrics 2012;130(3):397–406.
42. McKenna JJ, Bramley AM, Skarbinski J, et al. Pandemic influenza AVHIT: asthma in patients hospitalized with pandemic influenza A(H1N1)pdm09 virus infection-United States, 2009. BMC Infect Dis 2013;13:57.
43. Farne HA, Wilson A, Powell C, et al. Anti-IL5 therapies for asthma. Cochrane Database Syst Rev 2017;(9):CD010834.
44. Munitz A, Brandt EB, Mingler M, et al. Distinct roles for IL-13 and IL-4 via IL-13 receptor alpha1 and the type II IL-4 receptor in asthma pathogenesis. Proc Natl Acad Sci U S A 2008;105(20):7240–5.

45. Stier MT, Bloodworth MH, Toki S, et al. Respiratory syncytial virus infection activates IL-13-producing group 2 innate lymphoid cells through thymic stromal lymphopoietin. J Allergy Clin Immunol 2016;138(3):814–24.e11.

46. Cheung DS, Ehlenbach SJ, Kitchens RT, et al. Cutting edge: CD49d+ neutrophils induce FcepsilonRI expression on lung dendritic cells in a mouse model of postviral asthma. J Immunol 2010;185(9):4983–7.

47. Sigua JA, Buelow B, Cheung DS, et al. CD49d-expressing neutrophils differentiate atopic from nonatopic individuals. J Allergy Clin Immunol 2014;133(3): 901–4.e5.

48. Subrata LS, Bizzintino J, Mamessier E, et al. Interactions between innate antiviral and atopic immunoinflammatory pathways precipitate and sustain asthma exacerbations in children. J Immunol 2009;183(4):2793–800.

49. Khan SH, Grayson MH. Cross-linking IgE augments human conventional dendritic cell production of CC chemokine ligand 28. J Allergy Clin Immunol 2010; 125(1):265–7.

50. Tam JS, Jackson WT, Hunter D, et al. Rhinovirus specific IgE can be detected in human sera. J Allergy Clin Immunol 2013;132(5):1241–3.

51. Tam JS, Grayson MH. IgE and antiviral immune response in asthma. J Allergy Clin Immunol 2017;139(5):1717.

52. Bui RH, Molinaro GA, Kettering JD, et al. Virus-specific IgE and IgG4 antibodies in serum of children infected with respiratory syncytial virus. J Pediatr 1987; 110(1):87–90.

53. Rabatic S, Gagro A, Lokar-Kolbas R, et al. Increase in CD23+ B cells in infants with bronchiolitis is accompanied by appearance of IgE and IgG4 antibodies specific for respiratory syncytial virus. J Infect Dis 1997;175(1):32–7.

54. Aberle JH, Aberle SW, Dworzak MN, et al. Reduced interferon-gamma expression in peripheral blood mononuclear cells of infants with severe respiratory syncytial virus disease. Am J Respir Crit Care Med 1999;160(4):1263–8.

55. Metz G, Kraft M. Effects of atypical infections with Mycoplasma and Chlamydia on asthma. Immunol Allergy Clin North Am 2010;30(4):575–85, vii-viii.

56. Juhn YJ, Kita H, Yawn BP, et al. Increased risk of serious pneumococcal disease in patients with asthma. J Allergy Clin Immunol 2008;122(4):719–23.

57. Lehtinen P, Jartti T, Virkki R, et al. Bacterial coinfections in children with viral wheezing. Eur J Clin Microbiol Infect Dis 2006;25(7):463–9.

58. Webley WC, Salva PS, Andrzejewski C, et al. The bronchial lavage of pediatric patients with asthma contains infectious Chlamydia. Am J Respir Crit Care Med 2005;171(10):1083–8.

59. Denning DW, O'Driscoll BR, Hogaboam CM, et al. The link between fungi and severe asthma: a summary of the evidence. Eur Respir J 2006;27(3):615–26.

60. Specjalski K, Jassem E. Chlamydophila pneumoniae, Mycoplasma pneumoniae infections, and asthma control. Allergy Asthma Proc 2011;32(2):9–17.

61. Cunningham AF, Johnston SL, Julious SA, et al. Chronic Chlamydia pneumoniae infection and asthma exacerbations in children. Eur Respir J 1998;11(2):345–9.

62. Von HL, Vasankari T, Liippo K, et al. Chlamydia pneumoniae and severity of asthma. Scand J Infect Dis 2002;34(1):22–7.

63. Hahn DL, Schure A, Patel K, et al. Chlamydia pneumoniae-specific IgE is prevalent in asthma and is associated with disease severity. PLoS One 2012;7(4): e35945.

64. Smith-Norowitz TA, Silverberg JI, Kusonruksa M, et al. Asthmatic children have increased specific anti-Mycoplasma pneumoniae IgM but not IgG or IgE-

values independent of history of respiratory tract infection. Pediatr Infect Dis J 2013;32(6):599–603.

65. Nagayama Y, Tsubaki T, Nakayama S, et al. Bacterial colonization in respiratory secretions from acute and recurrent wheezing infants and children. Pediatr Allergy Immunol 2007;18(2):110–7.

66. Klemets P, Lyytikainen O, Ruutu P, et al. Risk of invasive pneumococcal infections among working age adults with asthma. Thorax 2010;65(8):698–702.

67. Bisgaard H, Hermansen MN, Buchvald F, et al. Childhood asthma after bacterial colonization of the airway in neonates. N Engl J Med 2007;357(15):1487–95.

68. Lim JH, Kim N, Lim SH, et al. Inverse relationship between helicobacter pylori infection and asthma among adults younger than 40 years: a cross-sectional study. Medicine (Baltimore) 2016;95(8):e2609.

69. Capili CR, Hettinger A, Rigelman-Hedberg N, et al. Increased risk of pertussis in patients with asthma. J Allergy Clin Immunol 2012;129(4):957–63.

70. Patel KK, Webley WC. Evidence of infectious asthma phenotype: chlamydia-induced allergy and pathogen-specific IgE in a neonatal mouse model. PLoS One 2013;8(12):e83453.

71. Horvat JC, Starkey MR, Kim RY, et al. Chlamydial respiratory infection during allergen sensitization drives neutrophilic allergic airways disease. J Immunol 2010;184(8):4159–69.

72. Morinaga Y, Yanagihara K, Miyashita N, et al. Azithromycin, clarithromycin and telithromycin inhibit MUC5AC induction by Chlamydophila pneumoniae in airway epithelial cells. Pulm Pharmacol Ther 2009;22(6):580–6.

73. Bacharier LB, Guilbert TW, Mauger DT, et al. Early administration of azithromycin and prevention of severe lower respiratory tract illnesses in preschool children with a history of such illnesses: a randomized clinical trial. JAMA 2015;314(19):2034–44.

Early Life Respiratory Syncytial Virus Infection and Asthmatic Responses

Catherine Ptaschinski, PhD[a], Nicholas W. Lukacs, PhD[b],*

KEYWORDS

- RSV • Asthma • Neonatal • Viral infections • Th2

KEY POINTS

- Early life development of the immune system is critical to control the long-term outcome of subsequent pulmonary responses, including asthma.
- The developing mucosal microbiome seems to control early respiratory viral responses that help to establish protective immune environments to avoid chronic pulmonary disease.
- Microbial and host metabolic responses help to shape the systemic immune responses through direct regulation of lung interaction and by influencing the bone marrow progenitor immune cell populations, possibly through epigenetic regulation.

INTRODUCTION

It is unclear whether early viral infections that induce significant airway disease are prognostic or causative for later airway obstructive disease and allergy, including the early development of asthma. The type of virus infection may not be as important as the timing and intensity of infection. Respiratory syncytial virus (RSV) infects nearly all infants by age 2 and is the leading cause of bronchiolitis in children worldwide. The Centers for Disease Control and Prevention estimate that up to 125,000 pediatric hospitalizations in the United States each year are due to RSV, at an annual cost of more than $300,000,000.[1] Although RSV is especially detrimental in very young infants whose airways are small and easily occluded, RSV has become recognized as an important pathogen in transplant recipients and the elderly, as well as patients with chronic lung disease including asthma and chronic obstructive pulmonary disease. Although anti-RSV antibodies are available and seem to alleviate severe disease,[2]

Disclosure Statement: The authors have nothing to disclose.
[a] Department of Pathology, University of Michigan Medical School, 109 Zina Pitcher Way, 4059 BSRB, Ann Arbor, MI 48109-2200, USA; [b] Mary H. Weiser Food Allergy Center, University of Michigan Medical School, 109 Zina Pitcher Way, 4059 BSRB, Ann Arbor, MI 48109-2200, USA
* Corresponding author.
E-mail address: nlukacs@umich.edu

Immunol Allergy Clin N Am 39 (2019) 309–319
https://doi.org/10.1016/j.iac.2019.03.002
0889-8561/19/© 2019 Elsevier Inc. All rights reserved.

they perform best when given prophylactically and to date few other options exist for combating the RSV infections in susceptible patient populations.[3–8] Several epidemiologic studies link severe RSV infection with the later development of hyperreactive airway disease that persists even years after the initial viral infection has resolved and increases the relative risk of developing asthma by 3- to 5-fold.[9–12] RSV has also been associated with asthma exacerbations and can cause prolonged episodes of illness.[13] It is likely that RSV and other viral infections drive an underlying immune phenotype,[14,15] with early disease with severe RSV as an independent variable for allergic asthma at age 7.[16]

The neonatal immune response is immature and evolutionarily skewed away from inflammatory responses in utero to avoid abortive birth.[17,18] At birth, the immune system must quickly mature and adapt to the new, nonsterile environment that includes both pathogenic and environmental stimuli. The initial responses are now thought to include significant influence by the commensal microbiome, wherein the gut seems to be most important[19] for both maturing the immune system and providing an appropriate tolerogenic environment. An early perturbation of the microbiome and/or pathogenic influence, such as viral and bacterial infections, may alter the normal/most appropriate progression of immune maturation. Previous studies with neonatal RSV infection have demonstrated that there are changes in the lung that include mucus production and increased immune cell populations that persist in the lung, including type 2 innate lymphoid cells that produce IL-5 and IL-13.[20,21] These responses during early life may be critical for the developing immune responses within the lung.

INNATE IMMUNE RESPONSES DURING RESPIRATORY SYNCYTIAL VIRUS INFECTION ESTABLISHES IMMUNE ENVIRONMENTS

It is important to understand the immune responses to RSV itself. In children with severe RSV infections, a number of leukocyte populations can be identified from airway samples, including neutrophils, macrophages, lymphocytes, and eosinophils.[22,23] Using animal models of disease to examine temporal expression of leukocyte accumulation, the initial cellular response within the first 4 days seems to consist of macrophages, neutrophils, and natural killer cell migration.[24,25] The differential activation of these cells may be important to establish an effective antiviral immune reaction and to avoid the adverse pathologic effects of the local response. The activation of CD4 and CD8 T cells depends on the "proper" activation of these innate cell populations.[26–29] A number of studies demonstrated that CD8+ T cells in mouse models of RSV disease do not properly clear virally infected cells.[26,30,31] Instead, it seems that the acquired immune response is shifted toward a Th2/Th17 immune environment that promotes a more pathogenic response.[32–35]

The innate immune system relies on the detection of patterns or conserved molecular motifs unique to various classes of pathogens, including viral nucleic acids that are either distinct in structure (dsRNA) or subcellular location (ssRNA). Toll-like receptors (TLRs) recognize different pathogen-associated molecular patterns and activate nuclear factor-κB and other innate signaling pathways including IRF3 that promote antiviral type I interferons (IFNs).[36–38] To transcribe and translate the protein components of RSV for assembly, the virus must go through a double-stranded RNA step. It is the recognition of this stage by a TLR (ie, TLR3) that likely leads to the recognition of the infection by the host immune response. The activation of TLR3 in dendritic cells (DC) leads to significant IL-12 and type I IFN production that is required for initiation of a cytotoxic IFNγ-mediated response.[39,40] TLR3$^{-/-}$ mice have an altered immune environment that is created and results in production of IL-13 leading to goblet cell metaplasia and mucus hypersecretion.[41] TLR7/TLR8 recognize ssRNA, whereas RIG-I, a cytoplasmic receptor, recognizes both ssRNA and dsRNA.[42-45] These innate molecules together can mediate the proper antiviral response by inducing type I IFN and IL-12, driving an appropriate antiviral response. In addition, these type 1 immune responses have been shown to diminish asthma responses by altering the local pulmonary immune environment. Therefore, by appropriately responding to the RSV responses with a Th1 phenotype, the immune environment of the lung is driven away from an asthmatic phenotype that allows the infant to avoid subsequent allergic responses. Again, it has been difficult to discern whether the initial viral responses promote the development of asthmatic disease or whether the host is predisposed to the allergic disease and responds inappropriately to the viral infection.

Early studies demonstrated that increased numbers of DC are recruited to the airway of asthmatics during severe disease and that corticosteroid treatment could control their recruitment.[46,47] Furthermore, studies in animal models indicated that DCs were required for the development of chronic eosinophil inflammation in the airway.[48] Although numerous DC subsets have now been identified, two of the major DC subsets are the CD11b[+], CD11c[+] myeloid/conventional DC (mDC/cDC) and CD11b[-], CD11c[+], B220[+], PDCA1[+] (mouse), CD123 (human), and Flt3[+] plasmacytoid DC (pDC).[49] CD103[+] DC are associated with the airway epithelium and also seem to play a role in the regulation of both early viral responses and asthmatic disease.[50,51] A series of studies have outlined distinct differences in the ability of DC subsets to induce responses. In particular, cDC have been implicated in driving a proallergic response,[52] whereas pDC have been identified to block or "tolerize" the pulmonary immune environment against Th2 responses,[53] either directly or indirectly through the activation of other cell populations.[54-57] RSV infection of DCs significantly alters the ability of mDC to express class II molecules and costimulatory molecules, preferentially express IL-10, and induce a Th1 response.[58-62] Thus, in the presence of an ongoing RSV infection, antigens (allergens) may induce a more skewed Th2 response owing to the alteration of DC subset activation. In our own laboratory and others, results have indicated that depletion of pDC from the lungs of RSV-infected mice results in a more pathologic response with increased airway hyperresponsiveness, mucus, and skewing toward Th2 cytokine profiles.[63] Studies have clearly established that both pDC and mDC subsets are recruited to the airway during RSV infection, and the severity of disease may depend on the numbers of each subset that respond to the stimulus along with the simultaneous level of exposure to allergen.[61,62,64,65] Understanding these responses may be most important during early life infections to begin to possibly promote an appropriate least pathogenic environment.

THE NEONATAL IMMUNE SYSTEM AND RESPIRATORY SYNCYTIAL VIRUS SUSCEPTIBILITY

The increased susceptibility of young infants to severe RSV is due in part to the functional immaturity of the neonatal immune system. The adaptive immune system does not begin to develop until after birth and takes several months to mature. Therefore, infants rely on the innate immune system early in life.[66] Although signaling through TLRs is relatively well-developed in neonates, the immune mediators that are activated by these signaling pathways are impaired in infants.[67,68] For example, IL-12, which is produced after RSV activation of TLR3, is one of the last cytokines to reach adult-like levels.[66] This lack of IL-12 early in life hinders the development of an appropriate Th1 response and likely contributes to skew the immune response toward a Th2 phenotype. Instead of IL-12, the innate response in infants is dominated by IL-23 and

IL-6 after TLR activation, leading to an enhanced Th17 response.[69] Although the research community often separates the Th2 and Th17 responses into separate categories, they are often produced in parallel in the most severe pulmonary disease phenotypes. The immaturity of the innate immune system may be an important driver of the Th2/Th17 phenotype and may predispose those infants with severe infection to develop childhood wheezing and subsequent asthma phenotypes.

Even though the neonatal immune system is not equipped to produce a strong Th1 response, the tolerogenic response in infants is well-developed. Neonatal immune cells produce high levels of IL-10 and transforming growth factor-β, correlating with an increase in the number and function of regulatory T (Treg) cells.[70,71] The immunosuppression provided by these cells is important for a number of reasons. They protect the developing fetus from the maternal immune system, they protect developing organs from inflammation, and they allow the microbiome to be established after birth.[19,72,73] Although these functions are critical for early life health and development, they also prevent the appropriate Th1 immune response from developing in response to RSV and other viral infections. These responses may perpetuate or drive the infant's immune response further toward an inappropriate pathogenic response.

EPIGENETIC MODIFICATIONS IN THE IMMUNE RESPONSE TO RESPIRATORY SYNCYTIAL VIRUS

Many of the differences observed between neonatal and adult immune function are due to epigenetic modifications that control inflammation and cytokine/mediator production. As mentioned elsewhere in this article, the infant immune system is poised toward Th2 effector function. Altered nucleosome remodeling in neonatal monocytes is linked with deficient DC development and impaired IL-12 production.[74] Although this lack of IL-12 impacts the differentiation of Th1 cells, there is another level of epigenetic changes in the CD4$^+$ T cells. Human neonatal CD4$^+$ T cells have increased methylation at the *IFNG* promoter, correlating with decreased IFN-γ production.[75] Furthermore, these cells are hypomethylated at the Th2 locus, leaving these cells in a poised state to produce Th2 cytokines.[76] Furthermore, a recent study from our group has found that premature infant cord blood monocytes are not poised to produce Th2 cytokines and have no activating histone H3K4 methylation marks in innate immune genes compared with full-term infants or adult monocytes, suggesting that the maturation of these responses occur around that time of birth at the latest stages of development.[77]

Infection with RSV itself can drive epigenetic changes in immune cells that can further alter immune function. We have previously found that RSV infection of DCs leads to altered histone methylation at promoter regions of proinflammatory cytokines, resulting in a decrease in the innate Th1-driving inflammatory response, and a subsequent skewing toward Th2 inflammation.[78] Other investigators have found that infection of bronchial epithelial cells drives changes in histone acetylation that results in altered innate immune function.[79] Furthermore, we have also described changes in histone modification in Treg cells[80] during RSV infection, demonstrating a role for epigenetic changes in multiple arms of the immune response to RSV. These changes, especially early in life, would have a lasting impact on a developing immune system that could skew the response toward a less favorable allergic/asthmatic phenotype.

MICROBIOME AND METABOLIC REGULATION OF IMMUNE RESPONSES

The effect of changes in the microbiome on allergic/asthmatic responses is a well-documented phenomenon that is associated with changes in the trajectory and development of immune responses, especially during infancy when the microbiome is initially established.[81–83] Studies in our laboratory have recently identified that early life infection in neonatal mice has a profound impact that changes the microbiome and metabolic profile that are coincident with the altered immune responses (unpublished data). Whether the changes in microbiome and metabolites are responsible for persistent immune changes is presently under investigation. Furthermore, infant cohort data indicate that it is the composition of the gut microbiome at 1 month of age that predicts the induction of multisensitization to allergens and the development of severe asthma later in life.[81] Recent studies on how microbiome-derived metabolites can regulate inflammation and immune responses have become an intense area of research. The concept that our immune system responses are influenced by environmental factors is important as a backdrop for understanding disease progression. Additionally, increases in a broad range of microbial- and/or mammalian-derived lipids, amino acids, and peptides with immunomodulatory potential support the growing concept that metabolic signaling may be an important mechanism by which the microbiome and host immune system interact.[84] Recent data have begun to build mechanistic evidence suggesting how the gut microbiome may regulate inflammation and immune responses. A link between diet and microbiome for the regulation of immune responses has been established with dietary fiber intake and presence of *Clostridiales* species. leading to production of short chain fatty acids and Treg cells.[85–88] Polyunsaturated fatty acids and short chain fatty acids together decrease adhesion molecule expression within tissues as well as cytokine levels by reducing inflammasome activation.[89–92] Our own recent work suggests that altering the microbiome by the addition of *Lactobacilli* promotes a favorable bacterial community, and gives rise to a diverse profile of lipid metabolites, including polyunsaturated fatty acids, which play a role in the regulation of immune responses.[93,94] These metabolites have both local effects on the barrier and systemic effects that promote immune response changes.

Metabolites from the microbiome can also drive epigenetic changes in the immune system through DNA methylation and histone modifications. short chain fatty acids from the microbiome both drive histone acetylation and inhibit histone deacetylation.[95] Furthermore, metabolites such as folate, butyrate, and acetate are important for DNA methylation.[96] Specifically, these metabolites promote Treg cells to maintain hyporesponsiveness to the commensal bacteria.[96] Together, it is rapidly becoming clear that the microbiome and its metabolic products are critical for antiviral responses and the perturbation of these communities can alter immune function to RSV and other viral responses as well as promoting a susceptible or resistant environment for the development of allergic asthmatic disease.

SUMMARY

It is becoming clear that our immune responses to environmental allergens and viruses that lead to altered lung function and asthmatic phenotypes are controlled by multiple interconnected mechanisms. These influences become even more profound early in life when the immune system is most susceptible to instruction, with many individuals genetically and/or environmentally predisposed to inappropriate immune responses. As shown in **Fig. 1**, the development of severe asthmatic disease may be due to numerous influences that likely begin in utero and continue to be influenced during early life. These can include the earliest influence of the developing microbiome as well as the influence of pathogens that drive altered immune responses, especially RSV that often infects infants early and can have a lasting influence on subsequent local lung

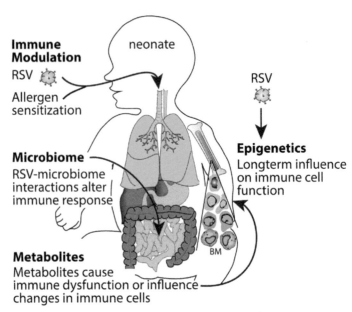

Fig. 1. Development of the early life immune system can be influenced by multiple environmental and pathogenic factors to drive allergen sensitization and asthma responses. RSV seems to be a contributory factor that can promote the development and severity of asthmatic disease. BM, bone marrow.

and perhaps systemic immune responses. The confluence of timing of the infection, the infants' environmental influences, as well as the development and stability of mucosal microbiome likely influence the genetic/epigenetic programming of the immune response. Together, these effects impact the development and severity of the subsequent asthmatic responses, but may also offer new areas to investigate novel and innovative interventions for blocking the development and/or treating asthmatic disease.

REFERENCES

1. Openshaw PJ, Dean GS, Culley FJ. Links between respiratory syncytial virus bronchiolitis and childhood asthma: clinical and research approaches. Pediatr Infect Dis J 2003;22:S58–64 [discussion: S64–5].
2. Carroll KN, Gebretsadik T, Escobar GJ, et al. Respiratory syncytial virus immunoprophylaxis in high-risk infants and development of childhood asthma. J Allergy Clin Immunol 2017;139:66–71.e3.
3. Centers for Disease Control and Prevention (CDC). Brief report: respiratory syncytial virus activity–United States, 2004-2005. MMWR Morb Mortal Wkly Rep 2005;54:1259–60.
4. Thompson WW, Shay DK, Weintraub E, et al. Mortality associated with influenza and respiratory syncytial virus in the United States. JAMA 2003;289:179–86.
5. Centers for Disease Control and Prevention (CDC). Respiratory syncytial virus activity–United States, 2000-01 season. MMWR Morb Mortal Wkly Rep 2002;51: 26–8.
6. Centers for Disease Control and Prevention (CDC). Respiratory syncytial virus activity–United States, 1999-2000 season. MMWR Morb Mortal Wkly Rep 2000;49: 1091–3.

7. Centers for Disease Control and Prevention (CDC). Update: respiratory syncytial virus activity–United States, 1998-1999 season. MMWR Morb Mortal Wkly Rep 1999;48:1104–6, 1115.

8. Pendl GG, Prieschl EE, Thumb W, et al. Effects of phosphatidylinositol-3-kinase inhibitors on degranulation and gene induction in allergically triggered mouse mast cells. Int Arch Allergy Immunol 1997;112:392–9.

9. Welliver RC. Review of epidemiology and clinical risk factors for severe respiratory syncytial virus (RSV) infection. J Pediatr 2003;143:S112–7.

10. Sigurs N, Gustafsson PM, Bjarnason R, et al. Severe respiratory syncytial virus bronchiolitis in infancy and asthma and allergy at age 13. Am J Respir Crit Care Med 2005;171:137–41.

11. Sigurs N. A cohort of children hospitalised with acute RSV bronchiolitis: impact on later respiratory disease. Paediatr Respir Rev 2002;3:177–83.

12. Sigurs N. Clinical perspectives on the association between respiratory syncytial virus and reactive airway disease. Respir Res 2002;3(Suppl 1):S8–14.

13. Hall CB, Long CE, Schnabel KC. Respiratory syncytial virus infections in previously healthy working adults. Clin Infect Dis 2001;33:792–6.

14. Lu S, Hartert TV, Everard ML, et al. Predictors of asthma following severe respiratory syncytial virus (RSV) bronchiolitis in early childhood. Pediatr Pulmonol 2016;51:1382–92.

15. Wu P, Hartert TV. Evidence for a causal relationship between respiratory syncytial virus infection and asthma. Expert Rev Anti Infect Ther 2011;9:731–45.

16. Simoes EA. RSV disease in the pediatric population: epidemiology, seasonal variability, and long-term outcomes. Manag Care 2008;17:3–6 [discussion: 18–9].

17. Ghazal P, Dickinson P, Smith CL. Early life response to infection. Curr Opin Infect Dis 2013;26:213–8.

18. Sharma AA, Jen R, Butler A, et al. The developing human preterm neonatal immune system: a case for more research in this area. Clin Immunol 2012;145:61–8.

19. Torow N, Marsland BJ, Hornef MW, et al. Neonatal mucosal immunology. Mucosal Immunol 2017;10:5–17.

20. Cormier SA, You D, Honnegowda S. The use of a neonatal mouse model to study respiratory syncytial virus infections. Expert Rev Anti Infect Ther 2010;8:1371–80.

21. Saravia J, You D, Shrestha B, et al. Respiratory syncytial virus disease is mediated by age-variable IL-33. PLoS Pathog 2015;11:e1005217.

22. Graham BS, Johnson TR, Peebles RS. Immune-mediated disease pathogenesis in respiratory syncytial virus infection. Immunopharmacology 2000;48:237–47.

23. Hogg JC. Childhood viral infection and the pathogenesis of asthma and chronic obstructive lung disease. Am J Respir Crit Care Med 1999;160:S26–8.

24. Hussell T, Openshaw PJ. IL-12-activated NK cells reduce lung eosinophilia to the attachment protein of respiratory syncytial virus but do not enhance the severity of illness in CD8 T cell-immunodeficient conditions. J Immunol 2000;165:7109–15.

25. Fawaz LM, Sharif-Askari E, Menezes J. Up-regulation of NK cytotoxic activity via IL-15 induction by different viruses: a comparative study. J Immunol 1999;163:4473–80.

26. Chang J, Srikiatkhachorn A, Braciale TJ. Visualization and characterization of respiratory syncytial virus F-specific CD8(+) T cells during experimental virus infection. J Immunol 2001;167:4254–60.

27. Mbawuike IN, Wells J, Byrd R, et al. HLA-restricted CD8+ cytotoxic T lymphocyte, interferon-gamma, and interleukin-4 responses to respiratory syncytial virus infection in infants and children. J Infect Dis 2001;183:687–96.

28. Aung S, Tang YW, Graham BS. Interleukin-4 diminishes CD8(+) respiratory syncytial virus-specific cytotoxic T-lymphocyte activity in vivo. J Virol 1999;73: 8944–9.
29. Tripp RA, Moore D, Jones L, et al. Respiratory syncytial virus G and/or SH protein alters Th1 cytokines, natural killer cells, and neutrophils responding to pulmonary infection in BALB/c mice. J Virol 1999;73:7099–107.
30. Chang J, Braciale TJ. Respiratory syncytial virus infection suppresses lung CD8+ T-cell effector activity and peripheral CD8+ T-cell memory in the respiratory tract. Nat Med 2002;8:54–60.
31. Chang J, Choi SY, Jin HT, et al. Improved effector activity and memory CD8 T cell development by IL-2 expression during experimental respiratory syncytial virus infection. J Immunol 2004;172:503–8.
32. Rey-Jurado E, Kalergis AM. Immunological features of respiratory syncytial virus-caused pneumonia-implications for vaccine design. Int J Mol Sci 2017;18 [pii: E556].
33. Mangodt TC, Van Herck MA, Nullens S, et al. The role of Th17 and Treg responses in the pathogenesis of RSV infection. Pediatr Res 2015;78:483–91.
34. Petersen BC, Dolgachev V, Rasky A, et al. IL-17E (IL-25) and IL-17RB promote respiratory syncytial virus-induced pulmonary disease. J Leukoc Biol 2014;95: 809–15.
35. Lambert L, Sagfors AM, Openshaw PJ, et al. Immunity to RSV in early-life. Front Immunol 2014;5:466.
36. Akira S, Hemmi H. Recognition of pathogen-associated molecular patterns by TLR family. Immunol Lett 2003;85:85–95.
37. Sandor F, Buc M. Toll-like receptors. I. Structure, function and their ligands. Folia Biol (Praha) 2005;51:148–57.
38. Roeder A, Kirschning CJ, Rupec RA, et al. Toll-like receptors as key mediators in innate antifungal immunity. Med Mycol 2004;42:485–98.
39. Kadowaki N, Ho S, Antonenko S, et al. Subsets of human dendritic cell precursors express different toll-like receptors and respond to different microbial antigens. J Exp Med 2001;194:863–9.
40. Spisek R, Bretaudeau L, Barbieux I, et al. Standardized generation of fully mature p70 IL-12 secreting monocyte-derived dendritic cells for clinical use. Cancer Immunol Immunother 2001;50:417–27.
41. Rudd BD, Smit JJ, Flavell RA, et al. Deletion of TLR3 alters the pulmonary immune environment and mucus production during respiratory syncytial virus infection. J Immunol 2006;176:1937–42.
42. Diebold SS, Kaisho T, Hemmi H, et al. Innate antiviral responses by means of TLR7-mediated recognition of single-stranded RNA. Science 2004;303:1529–31.
43. Heil F, Hemmi H, Hochrein H, et al. Species-specific recognition of single-stranded RNA via toll-like receptor 7 and 8. Science 2004;303:1526–9.
44. Lund JM, Alexopoulou L, Sato A, et al. Recognition of single-stranded RNA viruses by Toll-like receptor 7. Proc Natl Acad Sci U S A 2004;101:5598–603.
45. Yoneyama M, Kikuchi M, Natsukawa T, et al. The RNA helicase RIG-I has an essential function in double-stranded RNA-induced innate antiviral responses. Nat Immunol 2004;5:730–7.
46. Moller GM, Overbeek SE, Van Helden-Meeuwsen CG, et al. Increased numbers of dendritic cells in the bronchial mucosa of atopic asthmatic patients: downregulation by inhaled corticosteroids. Clin Exp Allergy 1996;26:517–24.

47. Jahnsen FL, Moloney ED, Hogan T, et al. Rapid dendritic cell recruitment to the bronchial mucosa of patients with atopic asthma in response to local allergen challenge. Thorax 2001;56:823–6.
48. Lambrecht BN, Salomon B, Klatzmann D, et al. Dendritic cells are required for the development of chronic eosinophilic airway inflammation in response to inhaled antigen in sensitized mice. J Immunol 1998;160:4090–7.
49. Webb TJ, Sumpter TL, Thiele AT, et al. The phenotype and function of lung dendritic cells. Crit Rev Immunol 2005;25:465–91.
50. Cui TX, Maheshwer B, Hong JY, et al. Hyperoxic exposure of immature mice increases the inflammatory response to subsequent rhinovirus infection: association with danger signals. J Immunol 2016;196:4692–705.
51. Munir S, Hillyer P, Le Nouen C, et al. Respiratory syncytial virus interferon antagonist NS1 protein suppresses and skews the human T lymphocyte response. PLoS Pathog 2011;7:e1001336.
52. Julia V, Hessel EM, Malherbe L, et al. A restricted subset of dendritic cells captures airborne antigens and remains able to activate specific T cells long after antigen exposure. Immunity 2002;16:271–83.
53. de Heer HJ, Hammad H, Soullie T, et al. Essential role of lung plasmacytoid dendritic cells in preventing asthmatic reactions to harmless inhaled antigen. J Exp Med 2004;200:89–98.
54. Yoneyama H, Matsuno K, Toda E, et al. Plasmacytoid DCs help lymph node DCs to induce anti-HSV CTLs. J Exp Med 2005;202:425–35.
55. Megjugorac NJ, Young HA, Amrute SB, et al. Virally stimulated plasmacytoid dendritic cells produce chemokines and induce migration of T and NK cells. J Leukoc Biol 2004;75:504–14.
56. Kohrgruber N, Groger M, Meraner P, et al. Plasmacytoid dendritic cell recruitment by immobilized CXCR3 ligands. J Immunol 2004;173:6592–602.
57. Hochrein H, Schlatter B, O'Keeffe M, et al. Herpes simplex virus type-1 induces IFN-alpha production via Toll-like receptor 9-dependent and -independent pathways. Proc Natl Acad Sci U S A 2004;101:11416–21.
58. Tripp RA, Moore D, Anderson LJ. TH(1)- and TH(2)-TYPE cytokine expression by activated t lymphocytes from the lung and spleen during the inflammatory response to respiratory syncytial virus. Cytokine 2000;12:801–7.
59. Bartz H, Buning-Pfaue F, Turkel O, et al. Respiratory syncytial virus induces prostaglandin E2, IL-10 and IL-11 generation in antigen presenting cells. Clin Exp Immunol 2002;129:438–45.
60. Bartz H, Turkel O, Hoffjan S, et al. Respiratory syncytial virus decreases the capacity of myeloid dendritic cells to induce interferon-gamma in naive T cells. Immunology 2003;109:49–57.
61. Kondo Y, Matsuse H, Machida I, et al. Regulation of mite allergen-pulsed murine dendritic cells by respiratory syncytial virus. Am J Respir Crit Care Med 2004; 169:494–8.
62. de Graaff PM, de Jong EC, van Capel TM, et al. Respiratory syncytial virus infection of monocyte-derived dendritic cells decreases their capacity to activate CD4 T cells. J Immunol 2005;175:5904–11.
63. Smit JJ, Rudd BD, Lukacs NW. Plasmacytoid dendritic cells inhibit pulmonary immunopathology and promote clearance of respiratory syncytial virus. J Exp Med 2006;203:1153–9.
64. Gill MA, Palucka AK, Barton T, et al. Mobilization of plasmacytoid and myeloid dendritic cells to mucosal sites in children with respiratory syncytial virus and other viral respiratory infections. J Infect Dis 2005;191:1105–15.

65. Silver E, Yin-DeClue H, Schechtman KB, et al. Lower levels of plasmacytoid dendritic cells in peripheral blood are associated with a diagnosis of asthma 6 yr after severe respiratory syncytial virus bronchiolitis. Pediatr Allergy Immunol 2009;20: 471–6.

66. Adkins B, Leclerc C, Marshall-Clarke S. Neonatal adaptive immunity comes of age. Nat Rev Immunol 2004;4:553–64.

67. Corbett NP, Blimkie D, Ho KC, et al. Ontogeny of toll-like receptor mediated cytokine responses of human blood mononuclear cells. PLoS One 2010;5:e15041.

68. Kollmann TR, Crabtree J, Rein-Weston A, et al. Neonatal innate TLR-mediated responses are distinct from those of adults. J Immunol 2009;183:7150–60.

69. Black A, Bhaumik S, Kirkman RL, et al. Developmental regulation of Th17-cell capacity in human neonates. Eur J Immunol 2012;42:311–9.

70. Hayakawa S, Ohno N, Okada S, et al. Significant augmentation of regulatory T cell numbers occurs during the early neonatal period. Clin Exp Immunol 2017;190: 268–79.

71. Rabe H, Lundell AC, Andersson K, et al. Higher proportions of circulating FOXP3+ and CTLA-4+ regulatory T cells are associated with lower fractions of memory CD4+ T cells in infants. J Leukoc Biol 2011;90:1133–40.

72. Mold JE, Michaelsson J, Burt TD, et al. Maternal alloantigens promote the development of tolerogenic fetal regulatory T cells in utero. Science 2008;322:1562–5.

73. Makhseed M, Raghupathy R, Azizieh F, et al. Th1 and Th2 cytokine profiles in recurrent aborters with successful pregnancy and with subsequent abortions. Hum Reprod 2001;16:2219–26.

74. Goriely S, Van Lint C, Dadkhah R, et al. A defect in nucleosome remodeling prevents IL-12(p35) gene transcription in neonatal dendritic cells. J Exp Med 2004; 199:1011–6.

75. White GP, Watt PM, Holt BJ, et al. Differential patterns of methylation of the IFN-gamma promoter at CpG and non-CpG sites underlie differences in IFN-gamma gene expression between human neonatal and adult CD45RO- T cells. J Immunol 2002;168:2820–7.

76. Rose S, Lichtenheld M, Foote MR, et al. Murine neonatal CD4+ cells are poised for rapid Th2 effector-like function. J Immunol 2007;178:2667–78.

77. Bermick JR, Lambrecht NJ, denDekker AD, et al. Neonatal monocytes exhibit a unique histone modification landscape. Clin Epigenetics 2016;8:99.

78. Ptaschinski C, Mukherjee S, Moore ML, et al. RSV-induced H3K4 demethylase KDM5B leads to regulation of dendritic cell-derived innate cytokines and exacerbates pathogenesis in vivo. PLoS Pathog 2015;11:e1004978.

79. Feng Q, Su Z, Song S, et al. Histone deacetylase inhibitors suppress RSV infection and alleviate virus-induced airway inflammation. Int J Mol Med 2016;38: 812–22.

80. Nagata DE, Ting HA, Cavassani KA, et al. Epigenetic control of Foxp3 by SMYD3 H3K4 histone methyltransferase controls iTreg development and regulates pathogenic T-cell responses during pulmonary viral infection. Mucosal Immunol 2015; 8:1131–43.

81. Fujimura KE, Sitarik AR, Havstad S, et al. Neonatal gut microbiota associates with childhood multisensitized atopy and T cell differentiation. Nat Med 2016;22: 1187–91.

82. Lynch SV. Gut microbiota and allergic disease. New insights. Ann Am Thorac Soc 2016;13(Suppl 1):S51–4.

83. Marsland BJ. Influences of the microbiome on the early origins of allergic asthma. Ann Am Thorac Soc 2013;10(Suppl):S165–9.

84. Li M, Wang B, Zhang M, et al. Symbiotic gut microbes modulate human metabolic phenotypes. Proc Natl Acad Sci U S A 2008;105:2117–22.
85. Zeng H, Chi H. Metabolic control of regulatory T cell development and function. Trends Immunol 2015;36:3–12.
86. Kosiewicz MM, Dryden GW, Chhabra A, et al. Relationship between gut microbiota and development of T cell associated disease. FEBS Lett 2014;588: 4195–206.
87. Geuking MB, McCoy KD, Macpherson AJ. Metabolites from intestinal microbes shape Treg. Cell Res 2013;23:1339–40.
88. Arpaia N, Campbell C, Fan X, et al. Metabolites produced by commensal bacteria promote peripheral regulatory T-cell generation. Nature 2013;504:451–5.
89. Teague H, Rockett BD, Harris M, et al. Dendritic cell activation, phagocytosis and CD69 expression on cognate T cells are suppressed by n-3 long-chain polyunsaturated fatty acids. Immunology 2013;139:386–94.
90. Draper E, Reynolds CM, Canavan M, et al. Omega-3 fatty acids attenuate dendritic cell function via NF-kappaB independent of PPARgamma. J Nutr Biochem 2011;22:784–90.
91. Narushima S, Sugiura Y, Oshima K, et al. Characterization of the 17 strains of regulatory T cell-inducing human-derived Clostridia. Gut Microbes 2014;5:333–9.
92. Borthakur A, Saksena S, Gill RK, et al. Regulation of monocarboxylate transporter 1 (MCT1) promoter by butyrate in human intestinal epithelial cells: involvement of NF-kappaB pathway. J Cell Biochem 2008;103:1452–63.
93. Fonseca W, Lucey K, Jang S, et al. Lactobacillus johnsonii supplementation attenuates respiratory viral infection via metabolic reprogramming and immune cell modulation. Mucosal Immunol 2017;10(6):1569–80.
94. Fujimura KE, Demoor T, Rauch M, et al. House dust exposure mediates gut microbiome Lactobacillus enrichment and airway immune defense against allergens and virus infection. Proc Natl Acad Sci U S A 2014;111:805–10.
95. Paul B, Barnes S, Demark-Wahnefried W, et al. Influences of diet and the gut microbiome on epigenetic modulation in cancer and other diseases. Clin Epigenetics 2015;7:112.
96. Obata Y, Furusawa Y, Hase K. Epigenetic modifications of the immune system in health and disease. Immunol Cell Biol 2015;93:226–32.

Importance of Virus Characteristics in Respiratory Syncytial Virus-Induced Disease

Homero San-Juan-Vergara, MD, PhD[a], Mark E. Peeples, PhD[b,c],*

KEYWORDS

- Respiratory syncytial virus (RSV) • Prefusion • Postfusion • G protein
- Neutralizing antibody • Vaccine • Genotypes

KEY POINTS

- The RSV attachment (G) glycoprotein and fusion glycoprotein, in its active pre fusion (pre-F) form, are responsible for virion attachment to target cells and entry by membrane fusion.
- Two RSV nonstructural proteins, NS1 and NS2, blunt the innate interferon antiviral response, its induction of an antiviral state in infected cells, and the adaptive immune response.
- The immune system responds to RSV infection by producing neutralizing antibodies primarily to the pre-F glycoprotein, which is therefore, the prime target of experimental vaccines.
- RSV disease is most severe and can be lethal in infants and in the elderly, influenced by immaturity or senescence of the immune system, underlying disease, and the RSV genotype.
- RSV infects the ciliated cells of the airway epithelium, inducing multiple mediators involved in allergy and asthma: CCL5, CXCL8, CCL2, CXCL10, and TSLP.

Respiratory syncytial virus (RSV) was discovered in 1955 in captive chimpanzees with symptoms of the common cold, and recognized as a human pathogen the following year.[1] In the 1960s, an ambitious plan to develop a vaccine using the same approach as the Salk killed polio vaccine was launched. RSV was grown in primary monkey

Disclosure Statement: M.E. Peeples has received research grants from NIH (nos. AI112524, AI095684, and AI093848), the Cystic Fibrosis Foundation, Janssen, and Pfizer, and fees for participation on an advisory board from ReViral and a lecture from Pfizer.
^a Division of Health Sciences, Fundación Universidad del Norte, Universidad del Norte, Bloque de Salud, Cuarto Piso 4-25L4, Km 5. Via Puerto, Barranquilla 081007, Colombia; ^b Center for Vaccines and Immunity, The Research Institute at Nationwide Children's Hospital, 700 Children's Drive, Columbus, OH 43205, USA; ^c Department of Pediatrics, The Ohio State University College of Medicine, Columbus, OH, USA
* Corresponding author.
E-mail address: mark.peeples@nationwidechildrens.org

Immunol Allergy Clin N Am 39 (2019) 321–334
https://doi.org/10.1016/j.iac.2019.04.001   immunology.theclinics.com
0889-8561/19/© 2019 Elsevier Inc. All rights reserved.

kidney cells, inactivated with formalin, and injected intramuscularly into children. The children were infected naturally during the usual "RSV season," between November and March. The control group had mild disease, whereas many of the immunized children required hospitalization, and 2 died.[2,3] It is thought that the killed vaccine established a Th2 inflammatory response pattern that exacerbated the disease rather than affording protection.[4]

The failure of the killed vaccine trial had a chilling effect on RSV vaccine work for nearly 40 years, with the group at the NIH, led by Robert Chanock, Peter Collins, and Brian Murphy, being the only group continuing the effort. Although we do not yet have an approved vaccine for RSV, in the past 10 years the NIH group has been joined by many others, and RSV vaccines are now on the horizon. Current approaches to RSV vaccines are described in more detail near the end of this review.

In the absence of a vaccine, an alternative approach was developed 20 years ago for the most "at risk" infants. Palivizumab (Synergis, MedImmune), a humanized monoclonal antibody (mAb), protected infants born prematurely or with cardiac malformations from severe RSV disease.[5] These infants represented ~50% of the severe RSV infections even though they represented less than 10% of the infant population. Palivizumab was successful in keeping these infants out of the hospital and, if not, at least out of the intensive care unit. The cost of palivizumab, however, is high and its use has been questioned on economic grounds.[6]

Severe RSV infection has been linked epidemiologically to wheezing and the development of asthma,[7] as described in other articles in this issue. To understand how RSV might contribute to atopy it is useful to understand some of what we have learned about RSV since its discovery 60 years ago, and what we still do not yet understand. This review highlights both.

FUNCTION OF VIRAL GLYCOPROTEINS: HOME INVASION

RSV is surrounded by a lipid envelope (**Fig. 1**), and uses it, like many viruses do, to enter a target cell by membrane fusion. The virion membrane is derived from the plasma membrane of the cell that produced the virion, and it fuses with the target cell membrane, becoming part of that cell's membrane. It sounds simple, but membranes do not readily fuse without some encouragement. Membrane fusion requires protein machinery: in the case of RSV, the attachment (G) glycoprotein binds the virion to the cell and the fusion (F) glycoprotein causes the lipid bilayers to merge. In immortalized cells, such as HEp-2, Vero, and HeLa, the G protein attaches to heparan sulfate proteoglycans (HSPGs).[8] The G protein is highly glycosylated (**Fig. 2**), but contains a central nonglycosylated region that includes a noose, held together by 2 closely spaced disulfide bonds.[9] The G protein is the least conserved of the RSV proteins, but N-terminal to the noose is a 13-amino acid strictly conserved region. C-terminal to the noose is a heparin-binding domain (HBD). The HBD is positively charged, enabling it to interact with the negatively charged heparan sulfate chains on cell surface HSPGs.[10]

Airway epithelial cells are difficult to examine in vivo but can be readily studied in well differentiated human airway epithelial (HAE) (or human bronchial epithelial [HBE]) cultures derived from donor tissue. RSV infects only the ciliated cells in these cultures (**Fig. 3**A), and only from the apical side.[11] HSPGs, the receptors on immortalized cells, are detected on the basal surface of the epithelium (**Fig. 3**B), but not on the apical surface[12] where RSV enters. Therefore HSPGs do not seem to be the RSV receptor on airway cells. Soluble HSPG competes with RSV infection of HEp-2 cells, but not infection of HAE. Conversely, a mAb (131-2g) against the

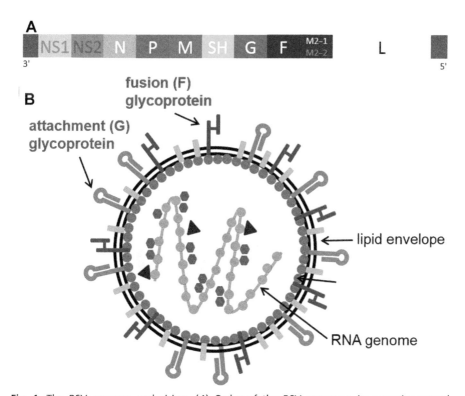

Fig. 1. The RSV genome and virion. (*A*) Order of the RSV genes on its negative strand genome. The viral polymerase begins at the 3′ end of the genome and transcribes each gene sequentially, releasing 10 capped, 5′ methylated and polyadenylated mRNAs. The gene colors match the colors of their protein in the virion depicted. The 3 genes colored gray are nonstructural genes that are found in infected cells, but not in the virion. (*B*) The negative single-strand RNA genome is covered by the nucleocapsid (N) protein, and associated with the phosphoprotein (P), the large (L) protein polymerase, and the M2-1 transcription antiterminator protein. The fusion (F) and attachment (G) glycoproteins are anchored in the lipid membrane, with the matrix (M) protein underlying the membrane. The 2 nonstructural (NS1 and NS2) and the M2-2 proteins (all colored *gray*) are not found in the virion. (*Courtesy of* S. M. Johnson, PhD, Ann Arbor, MI.)

G protein does not neutralize RSV in HEp-2 cells but does neutralize in HAE.[13] Together, these observations confirm that RSV uses a different receptor in HAE cultures than in immortalized cells.

The binding site for mAb 131-2g on the G protein is in the neck region of the cysteine noose (**Fig. 2**).[13] The third and fourth cysteines of the noose are separated by 3 amino acids, as are the cysteines found in fractalkine, the only member of the CX3C chemokine family.[14] Because this mAb blocks infection of HAE cultures by RSV, it suggests that this region of G, which is also close to the 13-amino acid absolutely conserved domain, is the region of the G protein that binds to its receptor. In the virus, removing 1 of these cysteines, or adding another amino acid between them, dramatically reduces infectivity in HBE cultures. It is possible that the fractalkine receptor, CX3CR1, might be a receptor for the RSV G protein on airway cells, and 3 groups have presented evidence consistent with this possibility.[13,15,16] However, a recent

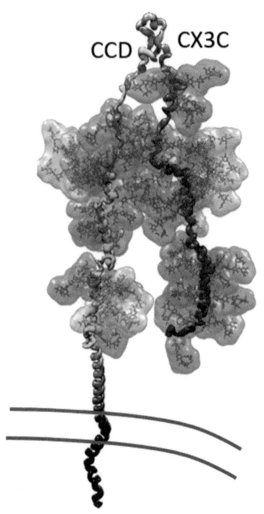

Fig. 2. Model of the RSV G protein. The G protein is anchored in the virion membrane near its N terminus and decorated with 3 to 7 N-linked glycans (*yellow*), depending on the strain, and 30 to 40 O-linked glycans (*gray*). The central region of G, likely to be at its apex, is the main unglycosylated portion of the G protein. This is the only portion of the G protein whose structure has been solved.[17,58,59] It contains a 13-amino acid sequence that is completely conserved in the G protein of all RSV strains, the central conserved domain (CCD), followed by a "cysteine noose" held together by 2 disulfide bonds. The 2 most downstream cysteines are separated by 3 amino acids, a motif similar to that used by the only CX3C chemokine, fractalkine. Fractalkine binds to its receptor, CX3CR1, which may also be the receptor for the RSV G protein on ciliated HBE cells.[13,15,16] The highly glycosylated domains flanking this central region are mucin-like, with many serines and threonines, the sites of O-glycan linkage. (*Adapted from* McLellan JS, Ray WC, Peeples ME. Structure and function of respiratory syncytial virus surface glycoproteins. Curr Top Microbiol Immunol 2013;372:83-104; with permission.)

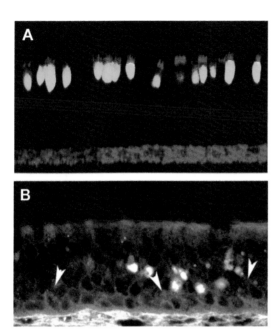

Fig. 3. RSV infects the apical multiciliated cells in HBE cultures. (*A*) Cross-section of HBE cultures infected with RSV-expressing GFP (*green*) and cilia (*red*). (*B*) Cross-section of uninfected HBE cultures stained with antibody to heparan sulfate (*pink*, indicated by *arrows*). (*From* [A] Zhang L, Peeples ME, Boucher RC, et al. Respiratory syncytial virus infection of human airway epithelial cells is polarized, specific to ciliated cells, and without obvious cytopathology. J Virol 2002;76(11):5658, with permission; and [B] Zhang L, Bukreyev A, Thompson CI, et al. Infection of ciliated cells by human parainfluenza virus type 3 in an in vitro model of human airway epithelium. J Virol 2005;79(2):1118; with permission.)

structural study of peptides from the G protein containing the cysteine noose suggests that the structure of the CX3C motif could not bind to a homolog of CX3CR1.[17] Two other potential RSV G protein receptors have been suggested from studies on immortalized cells: annexin II[18] and surfactant protein A.[19,20]

VIRUS-INDUCED MEMBRANE FUSION: SEALING THE DEAL

Once the G protein in the virion membrane binds to its receptor on the ciliated cell, the F protein takes over. The functional, prefusion (pre-F) protein is anchored in the virion surface membrane (**Fig. 4**). Pre-F protein monomers are cleaved twice in the Golgi by a furin-like protease to release a 27-amino acid peptide, pep27. The loss of pep27 allows 3 disulfide-linked F1-F2 monomers to coalesce into a fusion-active pre-F trimer, the functional form of the pre-F protein.[21] Pre-F is "metastable" meaning that it is easily, sometimes spontaneously, triggered to refold into its postfusion (post-F) form. In fact, some of the F protein on the virion surface is already in the spent, post-F form.[22]

F1 contains the transmembrane anchor at its C terminus, and the cleavage-generated, highly hydrophobic fusion peptide at its N terminus. The surface of the upper portion of pre-F is covered with the α helices, β sheets, and loops of F1. When the pre-F trimer is triggered, these structures refold into 1 very long α helix, with the fusion peptide at its N terminus, which inserts into the target cell membrane, provided that

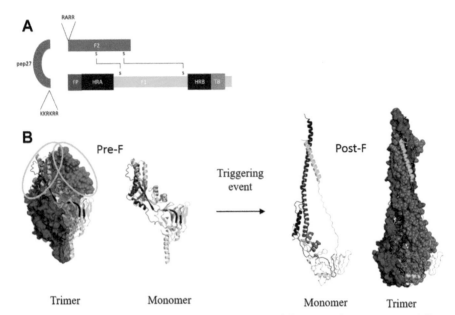

Fig. 4. RSV F protein cleavage products and structures of the F protein monomer and dimer in its pre-F and post-F forms. (*A*) F protein cleavage products. (*B*) Structures of the RSV pre-F and post-F proteins. Much of the apical portion of the pre-F head changes conformation when it is triggered (indicated by *yellow ellipses*), resulting in the post-F form. (*From* Hicks SN. Identification and Characterization of Essential Residues at the Apex of the RSV Fusion Protein. Dissertation, The Ohio State University 2017; with permission.)

the trimer is close enough to the target cell membrane. The virion G protein, binding the virion to the cell surface is likely responsible for that positioning before the pre-F protein is triggered, but is not directly involved in triggering pre-F. The smaller F2 fragment is an integral part of the head of the pre-F protein but does not move during the refolding of F1.[10]

It is not clear what triggers the F protein, but it seems likely that its interaction with a molecule on the cell surface, perhaps its own receptor or the lipid membrane, is responsible. Because RSV lacking its G protein is still infectious in immortalized cells, its F protein must be able to trigger on its own, without the aid of the G protein, and it likely has some attachment activity that positions it near the plasma membrane before triggering. Recently, the charged amino acids in the apical F2 loop were found to be essential for the fusion function of pre-F, further suggesting that F protein contact with the cell surface is critical for its triggering. Potential receptors for the F protein include nucleolin,[23] ICAM-I,[24] and the epidermal growth factor receptor.[25]

VIRION ASSEMBLY: GETTING IT ALL TOGETHER AND TAKING IT ON THE ROAD

The viral glycoproteins are produced and translocated into the rough endoplasmic reticulum where they receive their N-glycans: the G protein has 3 to 7 N-glycans (yellow clouds in **Fig. 2**); the F protein has 5 to 6 N-glycans, depending on the strain, but 2 to 3 of these are lost when pep27 is released from the F protein by cleavage in the Golgi. The G protein is also decorated with 30 to 40 O-linked glycans (gray clouds in **Fig. 2**). In fact, two-thirds of G's apparent molecular weight is due to sugars. In this way, the G protein resembles a mucin, highly glycosylated proteins abundant in the mucus that coats the surface of the airway epithelium. It is possible that this high glycan content on the surface of the virion may allow it to pass through the mucus layer and reach the underlying ciliated cells more easily.

The viral protein that orchestrates virion formation at the surface of infected cells is the matrix (M) protein. The M protein binds to nucleocapsids, the viral genome covered by N, and associated with the P, L, and M2-1 proteins. M also binds to the underside of cholesterol-rich domains in the plasma membrane that contain the G and F proteins.[26,27] The third viral membrane protein, SH (small hydrophobic), is also present on the cell surface and in virions. It has characteristics of a viroporin,[28,29] a channel that conducts ions through a membrane.[30] The SH protein has been shown to protect infected cells from attack by transforming growth factor α.[31] This complex of nucleocapsid and membrane, brought together by the M protein, buds outward from the plasma membrane to form new RSV virions.

AVOIDANCE OF THE INNATE IMMUNE RESPONSE: INTERFERON TAMPERING

Cells respond to most viral infections by producing a type I interferon (IFN) response. Three major routes—Toll-like receptor-3 (TLR3), retinoic acid-induced gene (RIG)-like helicase family of cytosolic DEXD/H box RNA helicases (RLR), and mitochondria-associated membranes—converge on the activation and consequent cytoplasmic-to-nuclear translocation of nuclear factor κB (NF-κB) and interferon regulator factor factors 3 and 7 (IRF-3/7), members of the interferon regulatory transcription factor family. In the nucleus, IRF-3 and NF-κB assemble respective transcriptional complexes that interact with the promoter regions of target genes, including IFN-β, IFN-λ1, and inflammatory cytokines. IFNs released from infected cells bind cognate receptors, which signal through activated STAT molecules to initiate transcription of interferon-stimulated genes ultimately responsible for establishing a cellular environment resistant to virus propagation. TLR3-dependent signaling that activates IRF3 kinases (IKKε and TBK1) via the adaptor protein TRIF, is triggered by TLR3 binding to double-stranded RNA motifs in the endosomes.

The RSV NS1 protein suppresses the cellular response to RSV replication, as demonstrated by the fact that A549 cells infected with ΔNS1-hRSV elicited a much more profound response than those infected with wt-hRSV.[32] Both the NS1 and NS2 proteins target RLR- and TLR3-dependent signaling at different levels. NS1 prevents RIG-I ubiquitination by competitively binding the C-terminal SPRY domain of TRIM25, which delivers the Lys 63-linked poly-ubiquitin moiety.[33] NS2 binds to the RIG-I CARD motif, preventing RIG-I from binding to MAVS,[34] impairing IFN-β production. NS1 associates with IRF3, thereby disrupting the transcriptional complex that IRF3 forms with CREB-binding protein, reducing its ability to bind to the IFN-β promoter.[35]

These inhibitory actions of NS1 and NS2 on type I IFN production may affect the way epithelial cells respond to infection by releasing proinflammatory cytokines and chemokines, which by themselves do not curtail RSV propagation. They can, however, create a Th-2-like environment conducive to the development of asthma and allergy. NS2-dependent NF-κB activation triggers the production of several immune response mediators, CCL5, CXCL8, CCL2, CXCL10, and TSLP.[36–39]

RSV infection induces interferon-α in the respiratory tract and systemically that decreases as RSV antigen levels and RSV disease recedes. But, compared with influenza virus, parainfluenza virus, or adenovirus, the levels of IFN-α in RSV-infected infants are low.[40] The lower levels of interferons may allow RSV to spread more widely in the respiratory tract. Because interferons also serve to enhance the adaptive immune response,[41–45] the ability of NS1 and NS2 to reduce the level of interferons during RSV infection likely contributes to the short-lived protective immunity. The adaptive immune response to RSV does not prevent periodic reinfection throughout life. In fact, RSV infection of elders is estimated to cause 14,000 deaths/y in the United States.[46]

The NS2 protein also mediates rounding and shedding of the RSV-infected epithelial cells.[47] These detached epithelial cells may contribute to the airway obstruction observed during bronchiolitis. NS2-mediated epithelial cell detachment could also contribute to allergic sensitization by disrupting the epithelial barrier function, which enhances Th2 polarization in asthma.[48]

INFECTION INDUCES PROTECTION: BUT NOT FOR LONG

The most effective RSV neutralizing antibodies bind the pre-F and not the post-F protein (see **Fig. 4**). Pre-F-specific antibodies bind regions whose structure changes when pre-F triggers. They probably inhibit pre-F triggering or refolding. As mentioned above, the apical surface of pre-F (antibody site φ) is critical for initiating fusion.[49] The lateral surface of pre-F (site V) also refolds to cause membrane fusion. Post-F binding antibodies, in general, are poorly neutralizing. Most post-F antibodies also bind to pre-F, in regions that are not disturbed by pre-F to post-F refolding. For example, palivizumab binds to both post-F and pre-F and is neutralizing, but at least 10-fold less so than pre-F-specific antibodies.[50] Antibody titers drop below protective levels over time, likely contributing to the ability of RSV to re-infect throughout life. Multiple reinfection suggest a poor memory B cell response. The appearance of CD8[+] T cells in the lungs correlates with clearance of RSV infection in adults experimentally infected with RSV.[51] But RSV infection activates mTOR mammalian target of rapamycin, which would impair CD8+ T-cell memory.[52]

RSV STRAIN DIFFERENCES: DO THEY ENABLE REPEAT INFECTIONS?

All RSV strains are categorized into 1 of 2 subgroups, A and B. Antibodies raised by infection with a group A virus will neutralize group B viruses, and vice versa, although 4- to 10-fold less efficiently. There are also many genotypes within each subgroup. Subgroup and genotype categorization are based on the sequence of the G gene because it is the least conserved of the RSV genes. The F protein is highly conserved (88% identical), but the G protein is not (48% identical). However, F and G gene variations segregate together in the phylogenetic tree and therefore have evolved together without the help of recombination.

It is possible that the diversity of RSV is at least partially responsible for the repeated infections with RSV that we experience throughout life. If so, the broad diversity of G sequences would suggest that the antibody response to G might be responsible. However, antibodies to the G protein are much less prevalent in serum and are responsible for only 1% to 10% of its neutralizing activity, both in immortalized cells and in HBE cultures.[53] Instead, antibodies to the much more highly conserved F protein are responsible for 90% to 99% of the neutralizing activity. Nevertheless, F antibodies induced by 1 RSV subtype neutralize the other subtype with reduced efficiency. Other likely reasons for repeated infections are that the overall immune response to an RSV infection is poor, that the response is short-lived, or that B-cell and/or T-cell memory is not efficiently established.

As mentioned above, RSV circulates each year within each community, but the strains from year to year are not random. Often the same A and the same B strains return for multiple consecutive years, then one or both will switch to a different strain the following year. The most likely explanation would seem to be that once a strain is established in a community, or in a region, it continues to smolder at a low level between RSV seasons. The number of cases increases again when the conditions are right, the following RSV season, until most susceptible people have been infected (herd immunity) and have some protection against that strain. Once individuals with some immunity to the strain that has been circulating for several years become the majority, a different strain would be more likely than the previous strain to infect and spread in that group.

RSV STRAIN DIFFERENCES: DO THEY AFFECT DISEASE SEVERITY?

Wheezing and asthma have been associated with severe RSV infections, as described elsewhere in this issue. Why are some infections severe but most are not? Certainly, some of the blame rests with the anatomy: the airways of the youngest infants are very small, and can be more easily occluded by excess mucus, cell debris, and inflammation. Some of the blame may also rest with the host response: suppression of the interferon response, as described in the previous section. But suppression of the interferon response could also be related to the RSV subgroup or strain causing the infection. In fact, RSV genotype A5 has recently been associated with disease severity,[54] as has the NA1 genotype.[55] The cause(s) of enhanced subgroup pathology is not known.

RSV continues to evolve. Two striking examples of this evolution are 2 strains that have arisen recently: RSV A Ontario (ON1) and RSV B Buenos Aires (BA), appeared in 1999 and 2010, respectively, and both have become the predominant strains of their subgroups in circulation. Both have a duplication (60 nucleotides for BA and 72 for ON1) in their G genes, in the C-terminal region of the G protein, but the duplicated sequences do not overlap. The explosive spread of both viruses in the population suggest that they have a major advantage over other strains in replication or spread. Because the only known role that the G protein plays in virus infection is attachment, the reason may be that their G proteins bind their receptor better. A comparison of RSV with and without the duplication found that the G protein did bind to cells better, but that did not translate to more rapid virus spread in an immortalized cell line.[56,57]

CURRENT VACCINE EFFORTS: THERE IS HOPE

A single vaccine is unlikely to be able to optimally protect all 3 age groups that need it: infants up to 6 months; young children 6 months to 5 years; and the elderly over 65 years. Infants younger than 6 months of age comprise ~60% of the severe RSV infections in childhood. These very young children are not able to respond to live attenuated vaccines for measles and mumps, viruses similar to RSV. Children 6 months to 5 years old comprise the remaining ~40% of severe infections. This group does respond to measles and mumps vaccine, although they respond better the older they are.

All infants receive antibody to RSV while in utero via active transport across the placenta, but the amount of antibody they receive depends on the titer of those antibodies in the mother. These transferred antibodies have a half-life of ~25 days in the infant, so by 4 months of age they drop to undetectable levels in nearly all infants. In an effort to protect these infants better and longer, one approach is to immunize pregnant women during their third trimester with an F protein vaccine so that more transplacental antibody will be transferred to the infant, protecting them longer, hopefully until they are at least 6 to 7 month old when they could be vaccinated effectively. At least 5 candidate F protein vaccines are currently in clinical trials in adults for eventual use in pregnant women, in the elderly, or both. One of these, a pre-F/post-F nanoparticle vaccine candidate (Novavax) is being tested in women of child-bearing age in a phase 3 clinical trial.

An alternative approach to immunizing pregnant women might be passive immunization with an antibody such as palivizumab. Monoclonal antibodies that specifically recognize the pre-F protein and are 10-fold better at neutralizing RSV than palivizumab are now available. One such pre-F antibody that has been modified to extend its half-life (MedImmune/Sanofi) is in phase 2 clinical trials. The goal is to administer this antibody once to the infant during the first month of life to provide protection for up to 6 months.

At 6 months, it may be possible to induce a more effective immune response in infants. A protein vaccine could be considered for infants. But because of the experience with the killed virus vaccine of the 1960s, which was also in essence a protein vaccine, there is a concern that it could suffer the same fate. However, it remains possible that other aspects of the killed vaccine such as the purity of the vaccine preparation used, may have caused the failure of that vaccine. Most groups are focusing on a live vaccine to stimulate an active immune response in the infant, but it could also be used to protect his/her older siblings from bringing RSV back from pre-school and his/her parents from passing on their "cold" to the infant (cocoon effect). Multiple live, attenuated RSV vaccines developed by NIAID are now in clinical trials (Sanofi, NIH).

Vectored vaccines are also being developed. Nonreplicating adenovirus expressing a stabilized version of the pre-F protein (Janssen) is being considered for immunization beginning at 2 months, at the same times as usual childhood vaccines. A Sendai virus-vectored stabilized pre-F vaccine, SeVRSV, is in phase 1 clinical trials (St. Jude/NIAID). An attenuated vaccinia virus, MVA, expressing 5 RSV proteins, is in phase 2 trials (Bavarian Nordic). A full list of RSV vaccine trials is maintained and updated by PATH as the "RSV Vaccine and mAb Snapshot" at their Web site: https://vaccineresources.org/search.php?q=RSV+Vaccines&cx=002645934641603553430%3Abilqaqmrhfo&cof=FORID%3A11&ie=UTF-8&sa=

FUTURE CONSIDERATIONS

Problems that remain to be solved include: protection of infants at the earliest times of life; protection against both RSV groups A and B; induction of long-lasting protection; and protection of the elderly who do not always respond well to vaccines. In addition to vaccines against RSV, there are several companies developing antiviral agents targeting the pre-F protein or the viral polymerase. Similar to any acute viral target, antiviral agents capable of reducing the severity and the length of the disease will be maximally useful in combination with rapid RSV diagnosis.

Progress toward effective RSV vaccines has been slow, but steady, supported by our growing understanding of how RSV works and how we respond to it. The pace of progress has improved dramatically over the past 10 years as more and more scientists and companies have joined the hunt. Several vaccine approaches are in clinical trials, with more on the horizon. Once we have a vaccine that efficiently prevents severe RSV disease, we will be able to determine how much of current allergy and asthma is caused by RSV infections early in life. It is hoped that this experiment will begin soon.

ACKNOWLEDGMENTS

The authors thank Will Ray, Sara Johnson, Stephanie Hicks, Supranee Chaiwatpongsakorn, Tiffany King, and Heather Costello for use of their graphics and insights. This work was supported by grants from the NIH (AI112524, AI095684 and AI093848 to M.E.P.) and from the Cystic Fibrosis Foundation (to M.E.P.), and from a Fulbright Fellowship (to H.S.-J.-V.).

REFERENCES

1. Chanock R, Roizman B, Myers R. Recovery from infants with respiratory illness of a virus related to chimpanzee coryza agent (CCA). I. Isolation, properties and characterization. Am J Hyg 1957;66(3):281–90.
2. Kapikian AZ, Mitchell RH, Chanock RM, et al. An epidemiologic study of altered clinical reactivity to respiratory syncytial (RS) virus infection in children previously vaccinated with an inactivated RS virus vaccine. Am J Epidemiol 1969;89(4): 405–21.
3. Prince GA, Curtis SJ, Yim KC, et al. Vaccine-enhanced respiratory syncytial virus disease in cotton rats following immunization with Lot 100 or a newly prepared reference vaccine. J Gen Virol 2001;82(Pt 12):2881–8.
4. Connors M, Giese NA, Kulkarni AB, et al. Enhanced pulmonary histopathology induced by respiratory syncytial virus (RSV) challenge of formalin-inactivated RSV-immunized BALB/c mice is abrogated by depletion of interleukin-4 (IL-4) and IL-10. J Virol 1994;68(8):5321–5.
5. IMpact-RSV. Palivizumab, a humanized respiratory syncytial virus monoclonal antibody, reduces hospitalization from respiratory syncytial virus infection in high-risk infants. The IMpact-RSV Study Group. Pediatrics 1998;102(3 Pt 1): 531–7.
6. Olicker A, Li H, Tatsuoka C, et al. Have changing palivizumab administration policies led to more respiratory morbidity in infants born at 32-35 weeks? J Pediatr 2016;171:31–7.
7. Sigurs N, Bjarnason R, Sigurbergsson F, et al. Asthma and immunoglobulin E antibodies after respiratory syncytial virus bronchiolitis: a prospective cohort study with matched controls. Pediatrics 1995;95(4):500–5.
8. Hallak LK, Collins PL, Knudson W, et al. Iduronic acid-containing glycosaminoglycans on target cells are required for efficient respiratory syncytial virus infection. Virology 2000;271(2):264–75.
9. Gorman JJ, Ferguson BL, Speelman D, et al. Determination of the disulfide bond arrangement of human respiratory syncytial virus attachment (G) protein by matrix-assisted laser desorption/ionization time-of-flight mass spectrometry. Protein Sci 1997;6(6):1308–15.
10. McLellan JS, Ray WC, Peeples ME. Structure and function of respiratory syncytial virus surface glycoproteins. Curr Top Microbiol Immunol 2013;372: 83–104.
11. Zhang L, Peeples ME, Boucher RC, et al. Respiratory syncytial virus infection of human airway epithelial cells is polarized, specific to ciliated cells, and without obvious cytopathology. J Virol 2002;76(11):5654–66.
12. Zhang L, Bukreyev A, Thompson CI, et al. Infection of ciliated cells by human parainfluenza virus type 3 in an in vitro model of human airway epithelium. J Virol 2005;79(2):1113–24.
13. Johnson SM, McNally BA, Ioannidis I, et al. Respiratory syncytial virus uses CX3CR1 as a receptor on primary human airway epithelial cultures. PLoS Pathog 2015;11(12):e1005318.
14. Tripp RA, Jones LP, Haynes LM, et al. CX3C chemokine mimicry by respiratory syncytial virus G glycoprotein. Nat Immunol 2001;2(8):732–8.

15. Chirkova T, Lin S, Oomens AG, et al. CX3CR1 is an important surface molecule for respiratory syncytial virus infection in human airway epithelial cells. J Gen Virol 2015;96(9):2543–56.

16. Jeong KI, Piepenhagen PA, Kishko M, et al. CX3CR1 is expressed in differentiated human ciliated airway cells and co-localizes with respiratory syncytial virus on cilia in a G protein-dependent manner. PLoS One 2015;10(6):e0130517.

17. Jones HG, Ritschel T, Pascual G, et al. Structural basis for recognition of the central conserved region of RSV G by neutralizing human antibodies. PLoS Pathog 2018;14(3):e1006935.

18. Malhotra R, Ward M, Bright H, et al. Isolation and characterisation of potential respiratory syncytial virus receptor(s) on epithelial cells. Microbes Infect 2003;5(2): 123–33.

19. Barr FE, Pedigo H, Johnson TR, et al. Surfactant protein-A enhances uptake of respiratory syncytial virus by monocytes and U937 macrophages. Am J Respir Cell Mol Biol 2000;23(5):586–92.

20. Hickling TP, Malhotra R, Bright H, et al. Lung surfactant protein A provides a route of entry for respiratory syncytial virus into host cells. Viral Immunol 2000;13(1): 125–35.

21. Gilman MS, Moin SM, Mas V, et al. Characterization of a prefusion-specific antibody that recognizes a quaternary, cleavage-dependent epitope on the RSV fusion glycoprotein. PLoS Pathog 2015;11(7):e1005035.

22. Liljeroos L, Krzyzaniak MA, Helenius A, et al. Architecture of respiratory syncytial virus revealed by electron cryotomography. Proc Natl Acad Sci U S A 2013; 110(27):11133–8.

23. Tayyari F, Marchant D, Moraes TJ, et al. Identification of nucleolin as a cellular receptor for human respiratory syncytial virus. Nat Med 2011;17(9):1132–5.

24. Behera AK, Matsuse H, Kumar M, et al. Blocking intercellular adhesion molecule-1 on human epithelial cells decreases respiratory syncytial virus infection. Biochem Biophys Res Commun 2001;280(1):188–95.

25. Currier MG, Lee S, Stobart CC, et al. EGFR Interacts with the fusion protein of respiratory syncytial virus strain 2-20 and mediates infection and mucin expression. PLoS Pathog 2016;12(5):e1005622.

26. Ludwig A, Nguyen TH, Leong D, et al. Caveolae provide a specialized membrane environment for respiratory syncytial virus assembly. J Cell Sci 2017;130(6): 1037–50.

27. San-Juan-Vergara H, Sampayo-Escobar V, Reyes N, et al. Cholesterol-rich microdomains as docking platforms for respiratory syncytial virus in normal human bronchial epithelial cells. J Virol 2012;86(3):1832–43.

28. Araujo GC, Silva RH, Scott LP, et al. Structure and functional dynamics characterization of the ion channel of the human respiratory syncytial virus (hRSV) small hydrophobic protein (SH) transmembrane domain by combining molecular dynamics with excited normal modes. J Mol Model 2016;22(12):286.

29. Li Y, To J, Verdia-Baguena C, et al. Inhibition of the human respiratory syncytial virus small hydrophobic protein and structural variations in a bicelle environment. J Virol 2014;88(20):11899–914.

30. Heminway BR, Yu Y, Tanaka Y, et al. Analysis of respiratory syncytial virus F, G, and SH proteins in cell fusion. Virology 1994;200(2):801–5.

31. Fuentes S, Tran KC, Luthra P, et al. Function of the respiratory syncytial virus small hydrophobic protein. J Virol 2007;81(15):8361–6.

32. Hastie ML, Headlam MJ, Patel NB, et al. The human respiratory syncytial virus nonstructural protein 1 regulates type I and type II interferon pathways. Mol Cell Proteomics 2012;11(5):108–27.
33. Ban J, Lee NR, Lee NJ, et al. Human respiratory syncytial virus NS 1 targets TRIM25 to suppress RIG-I ubiquitination and subsequent RIG-I-mediated antiviral signaling. Viruses 2018;10(12) [pii:E716].
34. Ling Z, Tran KC, Teng MN. Human respiratory syncytial virus nonstructural protein NS2 antagonizes the activation of beta interferon transcription by interacting with RIG-I. J Virol 2009;83(8):3734–42.
35. Ren J, Liu T, Pang L, et al. A novel mechanism for the inhibition of interferon regulatory factor-3-dependent gene expression by human respiratory syncytial virus NS1 protein. J Gen Virol 2011;92(Pt 9):2153–9.
36. Spann KM, Tran KC, Collins PL. Effects of nonstructural proteins NS1 and NS2 of human respiratory syncytial virus on interferon regulatory factor 3, NF-kappaB, and proinflammatory cytokines. J Virol 2005;79(9):5353–62.
37. Lay MK, Gonzalez PA, Leon MA, et al. Advances in understanding respiratory syncytial virus infection in airway epithelial cells and consequential effects on the immune response. Microbes Infect 2013;15(3):230–42.
38. Machado D, Pizzorno A, Hoffmann J, et al. Role of p53/NF-kappaB functional balance in respiratory syncytial virus-induced inflammation response. J Gen Virol 2018;99(4):489–500.
39. Bueno SM, Gonzalez PA, Pacheco R, et al. Host immunity during RSV pathogenesis. Int Immunopharmacol 2008;8(10):1320–9.
40. Nakayama T, Sonoda S, Urano T, et al. Detection of alpha-interferon in nasopharyngeal secretions and sera in children infected with respiratory syncytial virus. Pediatr Infect Dis J 1993;12(11):925–9.
41. Kim D, Niewiesk S. Synergistic induction of interferon alpha through TLR-3 and TLR-9 agonists stimulates immune responses against measles virus in neonatal cotton rats. Vaccine 2014;32(2):265–70.
42. Gans HA. The status of live viral vaccination in early life. Vaccine 2013;31(21):2531–7.
43. Pulendran B, Ahmed R. Translating innate immunity into immunological memory: implications for vaccine development. Cell 2006;124(4):849–63.
44. Pulendran B, Ahmed R. Immunological mechanisms of vaccination. Nat Immunol 2011;12(6):509–17.
45. Tough DF. Modulation of T-cell function by type I interferon. Immunol Cell Biol 2012;90(5):492–7.
46. Walsh EE, Falsey AR. Respiratory syncytial virus infection in adult populations. Infect Disord Drug Targets 2012;12(2):98–102.
47. Liesman RM, Buchholz UJ, Luongo CL, et al. RSV-encoded NS2 promotes epithelial cell shedding and distal airway obstruction. J Clin Invest 2014;124(5):2219–33.
48. Georas SN, Rezaee F. Epithelial barrier function: at the front line of asthma immunology and allergic airway inflammation. J Allergy Clin Immunol 2014;134(3):509–20.
49. Hicks SN, Chaiwatpongsakorn S, Costello HM, et al. Five residues in the apical loop of the respiratory syncytial virus fusion protein F2 subunit are critical for its fusion activity. J Virol 2018;92(15) [pii:e00621-18].
50. McLellan JS, Chen M, Leung S, et al. Structure of RSV fusion glycoprotein trimer bound to a prefusion-specific neutralizing antibody. Science 2013;340(6136):1113–7.

51. Jozwik A, Habibi MS, Paras A, et al. RSV-specific airway resident memory CD8+ T cells and differential disease severity after experimental human infection. Nat Commun 2015;6:10224.
52. de Souza AP, de Freitas DN, Antuntes Fernandes KE, et al. Respiratory syncytial virus induces phosphorylation of mTOR at ser2448 in CD8 T cells from nasal washes of infected infants. Clin Exp Immunol 2016;183(2):248–57.
53. Ngwuta JO, Chen M, Modjarrad K, et al. Prefusion F-specific antibodies determine the magnitude of RSV neutralizing activity in human sera. Sci Transl Med 2015;7(309):309ra162.
54. Rodriguez-Fernandez R, Tapia LI, Yang CF, et al. Respiratory syncytial virus genotypes, host immune profiles, and disease severity in young children hospitalized with bronchiolitis. J Infect Dis 2017;217(1):24–34.
55. Midulla F, Nenna R, Scagnolari C, et al. How respiratory syncytial virus genotypes influence the clinical course in infants hospitalized for bronchiolitis. J Infect Dis 2019;219(4):526–34.
56. Hotard AL, Laikhter E, Brooks K, et al. Functional analysis of the 60-nucleotide duplication in the respiratory syncytial virus buenos aires strain attachment glycoprotein. J Virol 2015;89(16):8258–66.
57. Johnson SM. Respiratory syncytial virus uses CX3CR1 as a cellular receptor on primary human airway epithelial cultures [Dissertation]. Columbus (OH): The Ohio State University; 2015.
58. Fedechkin SO, George NL, Wolff JT, et al. Structures of respiratory syncytial virus G antigen bound to broadly neutralizing antibodies. Sci Immunol 2018;3(21) [pii:eaar3534].
59. McLellan JS, Yang Y, Graham BS, et al. Structure of respiratory syncytial virus fusion glycoprotein in the postfusion conformation reveals preservation of neutralizing epitopes. J Virol 2011;85(15):7788–96.

Rhinovirus and Asthma Exacerbations

Joshua L. Kennedy, MD[a,b,c,]*, Sarah Pham, MD[a], Larry Borish, MD[d,e,f]

KEYWORDS

- Allergy • Asthma • Genetics • IgE • Rhinovirus

KEY POINTS

- Most asthma exacerbations in children and adolescents are associated with development of a rhinovirus (RV) infection.
- These RV-mediated exacerbations seem to require concomitant exposure to a bystander allergen to which the asthmatic is highly sensitized.
- Asthmatics can be genetically prone to RV-mediated exacerbations.
- Targeting IgE and type 2 inflammation–promoting cytokines can mitigate the likelihood of developing RV-induced asthma exacerbations.

INTRODUCTION

Asthma is an increasing public health concern with more than 8% of children and adults now having this condition.[1,2] Asthma exacerbations, or loss of symptom control that includes increased cough, wheezing, and difficulty breathing, provide the

Disclosures: J.L. Kennedy and his laboratory are supported by the NIH (K08AI121345, UL1TR000039, KL2TR000063, P20GM121293), the Centers for Translational Science Award Western Consortium Grant, Arkansas Children's Research Institute Marion B. Lyon New Scientist Career Development Award, and the Arkansas Biosciences Institute. S. Pham reports no conflicts of interest. L. Borish does consulting work for Novartis, Teva, Astra Zeneca, and Regeneron. His laboratory at the University of Virginia receives research grants from the NIH and from Astra Zeneca.

[a] Department of Pediatrics, University of Arkansas for Medical Sciences, 13 Children's Way, Slot 512-13, Little Rock, AR 72202, USA; [b] Department of Internal Medicine, University of Arkansas for Medical Sciences, 13 Children's Way, Slot 512-13, Little Rock, AR 72202, USA; [c] Arkansas Children's Research Institute, University of Arkansas for Medical Sciences, 13 Children's Way, Slot 512-13, Little Rock, AR 72202, USA; [d] Department of Medicine, University of Virginia Health Systems, MR4 Building Room 5041, 409 Lane Road, Charlottesville, VA 22903, USA; [e] Department of Microbiology, University of Virginia Health Systems, MR4 Building Room 5041, 409 Lane Road, Charlottesville, VA 22903, USA; [f] Carter Immunology Center, University of Virginia Health Systems, MR4 Building Room 5041, 409 Lane Road, Charlottesville, VA 22903, USA
* Corresponding author. University of Arkansas for Medical Sciences, 13 Children's Way, Slot 512-13, Little Rock, AR 72202.
E-mail address: kennedyjoshual@uams.edu

greatest morbidity to asthmatics and can lead to hospitalizations and, rarely, to death. Importantly, in 2016, ~54% of children[2] and ~45% of adults[1] with a diagnosis of current asthma reported having 1 or more asthma exacerbations. Although an exact mechanism/causal relationship is not clear, rhinovirus (RV) infections have been extensively linked to asthma exacerbations. From 60% to 80% of children with asthma exacerbations seen in the emergency department (ED) have a concomitant RV infection.[3,4]

This article evaluates the evidence regarding the association of RV infections with asthma exacerbations. Further, it examines the effects of genetic polymorphisms on the generation of viral-induced asthma exacerbations and discusses the role of the atopic host in the relationship between exacerbations and RV infections. Because of the overwhelming evidence linking RV infection and asthma exacerbations, the ultimate goal is to gather potential mechanisms concerning how this virus can cause such chaos in asthmatics and to speculate on potential therapeutics that may improve outcomes in the future.

THE EVIDENCE THAT RHINOVIRUS INFECTION CAUSES ASTHMA EXACERBATIONS

Viral respiratory infections are the most common triggers for exacerbations of asthma, with human RV, particularly subtypes A and C, being the most frequent.[5] Hospital admission rates for asthma exacerbations in school-aged children correlate with the seasonal increase of RV infections in the fall and again in the spring, with similar peaks observed in adults.[6] However, RV infections are ubiquitous and can occur throughout the year. Many of these infections do not cause exacerbations, and some remain completely asymptomatic.[7] This lack of a consistent association has led to a debate as to whether RV infection is causal or is merely associated in asthma exacerbations.

The Con: Rhinovirus Is Associated with Asthma Exacerbations

In the context of asthma exacerbations, there is ongoing debate as to whether RV infections are the sole cause, are synergistic with other factors, or are merely associated with exacerbations. For example, studies have detected the presence of RV in patients who are asymptomatic or have minimal symptoms. In one prospective study, 126 infants were followed for the first 2 years of life.[8] Among these subjects, RV was the most predominant virus detected, regardless of the presence of symptoms. In the Early Unbiased Risk Assessment of Pediatric Asthma (EUROPA) prospective case-control follow-up study, 140 symptomatic and 96 asymptomatic children were selected from a birth cohort and were followed for 3 years (November 2009 through December 2012).[9] RV-A and RV-C were detected with similar prevalence between symptomatic (which included both wheezing and nonwheezing children) and control children. Of note, RV-B was detected significantly more in the control group.[9] Improved detection techniques using polymerase chain reaction (PCR) and more regular screening may lead to recognition of an even greater prevalence of indolent RV infection in the asymptomatic population.

When examining RV infections in the setting of experimental challenge models, studies have suggested that RV may not cause asthma exacerbations. In one of the first studies to examine this, 21 adult asthmatics were exposed to RV,[10] and their symptoms, spirometry measurements, and histamine challenges were assessed before RV exposure, daily while symptomatic, and 3 weeks post-RV exposure. The results showed no significant changes in spirometry or histamine sensitivity, either as a whole group or when subcategorized by asthma severity.

The Pro: Rhinovirus Causes Asthma Exacerbations

In contrast, many other studies have shown a causal relationship between exposure to RV and asthma exacerbations or, alternatively, objective evidence of increased airways hyperresponsiveness (AHR). In a prospective study following subjects from the same household, 1 with asthma and 1 without, subjects had similar frequency of RV infections, although the asthmatics developed greater lower respiratory symptoms during the infection.[11,12] Other studies have shown increased susceptibility and symptoms, specifically during RV-C infections in children with asthma. For example, in one study, the frequency of RV-C infections was much higher in the asthma population than in the community as a whole, suggesting that asthmatic children are more susceptible to infection with RV-C. The same study showed that subjects with RV-C had higher asthma severity scores than children with RV-A or RV-B.[13]

More direct evidence of a causative role of RV in acute exacerbations of asthma has been established in the experimental RV infection model.[14–16] In a study by Zambrano and colleagues,[14] patients with asthma and high total immunoglobulin (Ig) E levels (>371 IU/mL) infected with RV-A16 had increased methacholine sensitivity by day 4 of the study, and that increase remained evident through day 21. These subjects experienced significantly worse lower respiratory symptoms than their control counterparts. Another experimental infection study exposed subjects with asthma on inhaled corticosteroids (ICS) to RV-A16. Subjects had increased symptoms with a mean period between peak cold and peak asthma symptoms of 2.1 (0.3–3.9) days.[15] There was also increased β-agonist use, suggesting loss of symptom control; however, these asthmatics did not experience a reduction in lung function postinoculation. The investigators suggest that long-term ICS use might inhibit this process. In a more recent study, 10 adult atopic asthmatics and 15 controls were infected with RV-A16[16] and bronchial biopsies were taken at 14 days before infection, 4 days after, and 6 weeks postinfection. There were no significant differences in the number of neutrophils at baseline between asthmatics and controls. In asthmatics, the change in number of epithelial and subepithelial neutrophils from baseline to day 4 was significantly higher. Those asthmatics who had higher epithelial neutrophil counts had a significantly larger decrease in forced expiratory volume in 1 second postinfection.

Recently, in vitro studies of human precision-cut lung slices (PCLS) from 7 asthmatics and 9 control lungs infected with RV-A39 showed increased AHR (asthma mean, 35% change in AHR after infection; nonasthma mean, 17.7% change in AHR after infection; $P<.05$)[17](**Fig. 1**A). These studies also found differences in the inflammatory responses generated by asthmatic tissue compared with controls, specifically related to type 2 (T2) inflammation in the asthmatic tissue, which is discussed further later. To our knowledge, this study is the first to show direct evidence of AHR to RV in asthma tissue ex vivo.

GENETIC SUSCEPTIBILITIES LEADING TO ASTHMA EXACERBATIONS AS RELATED TO RHINOVIRUS INFECTION

Although it may be difficult to connect genetic predisposition with a future outcome such as asthma exacerbation risk, researchers have recently shed light on mechanisms whereby this might be the case. Specifically, several candidate genes have been identified that provide potential associations between genetic polymorphisms and viral respiratory illness outcomes, including asthma exacerbations. Some of these genes (eg, *STAT4, JAK2, MX1, VDR, DDX58,* and *EIF2AK2*) are important in antiviral and innate immune responses and, as such, might impart susceptibility to respiratory viruses, increase infection severity, and lead to virus-induced asthma exacerbations.[18,19]

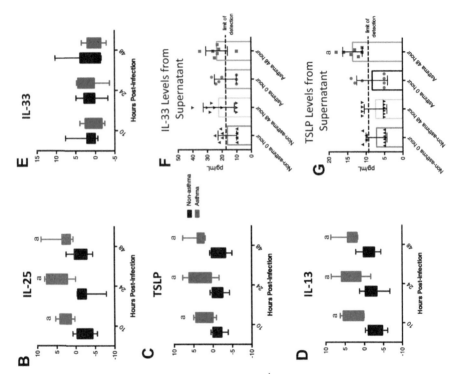

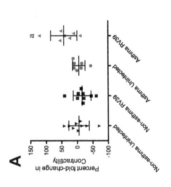

Studies have highlighted the importance of one particular gene in contributing to RV-induced asthma exacerbations: the genetic variant of the transmembrane protein cadherin-related family members 3 (*CDHR3*), which has been identified as the RV-C receptor.[20] In a Swedish study, 122 wheezing subjects and 94 controls (ages 6–48 months) were seen both during acute episodes for wheeze and at a follow-up visit 2 to 3 months later.[21] The genotype AA/AG at the *CDHR3* gene was significantly overrepresented in wheezing children; moreover, children with this genotype sought emergency care because of respiratory symptoms at a significantly higher rate. The AA/AG genetic variant results in an amino acid change (Cys529Tyr) in the CDHR3 protein, at a site that is associated with increased binding, internalization, and subsequent replication of RV-C strains. As such, these findings suggest a mechanism for greater susceptibility to, and symptoms during, RV-C infection that could drive exacerbations of asthma. The same outcome of this *CDHR3* gene mutation was replicated in early-onset asthmatics in a different population. In this retrospective study of 2 cohorts (distinguished by geographic location: 967 healthy and 814 asthmatic adults in Tsukuba and 994 healthy and 591 asthmatic adults in Hokkaido), a greater number of early-onset asthmatics ($\leq$10 years of age) had the A (Cys529Tyr) allele.[22] When only atopic individuals from both cohorts were examined, the association between the *CDHR3* variant and early-onset asthma reached significance. These findings tie together the importance of genetic susceptibility to RV infection in combination with allergy (and by extension T2 status) in the generation of asthma exacerbations.

THE ROLE OF ALLERGY IN RHINOVIRUS-ASSOCIATED ASTHMA EXACERBATIONS

As mentioned, 60% to 80% of children who are seen for asthma exacerbations have a concomitant RV infection[3,4]; however, almost all (ie, $\geq$85%) are also allergic.[23] It is reasonable to speculate that transient increases in exposure to allergen are not a convincing explanation of most attacks. However, almost all the evidence regarding the effects of RV relates primarily to allergic patients. In a study of Costa Rican children, the relationship of dust mite allergy and severe asthma exacerbations in the context of RV infection was positively correlated.[24] Ninety-six acutely wheezing children, 65 stable asthmatics, and 126 controls were enrolled through the ED. Multiple allergen-specific IgE antibodies were measured, and IgE to dust mite (*Dermatophagoides pteronyssinus*, *Dermatophagoides farinae*, or *Blomia tropicalis*) allergens were the most commonly detected. In this population, the probability of acute wheezing was significantly associated with increasing IgE titers to dust mite, and this probability substantially increased if the subject was RV positive during the exacerbation (**Fig. 2**, **Table 1**). These data produced a remarkable positive odds ratio of 30

◄————————————————————————————————

Fig. 1. RV39 infection of human PCLS from asthma donors. (*A*) Comparison of carbachol (CCh)-induced airway responsiveness in donors with and without asthma before and after infection with RV39. RV39 infection causes airway hyperresponsiveness to CCh only in PCLS from donors with a history of asthma. (*B–E*) Interleukin (IL)-25, TSLP, IL-13, and IL-33 gene expression from RV39-infected PCLS. There are significant increases in the expression of IL-25, TSLP, and IL-13 in the PCLS from asthma donors compared with controls without asthma. (*F, G*) IL-33 and TSLP protein levels in supernatants from RV39-infected PCLS in donors with and without asthma. There are significantly increased TSLP protein levels in those donors with a history of asthma after infection with RV39. [a] $P<.05$. mRNA, messenger RNA. (*Adapted from* Kennedy JL, Koziol-White CJ, Jeffus S, et al. Effects of rhinovirus 39 infection on airway hyperresponsiveness to carbachol in human airways precision cut lung slices. J Allergy Clin Immunol 2018;141(5):1888; with permission.)

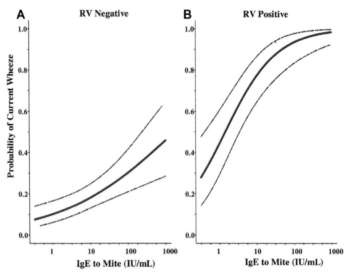

Fig. 2. Probability of current wheezing based on increasing titers of IgE to *D pteronyssinus* in children with (*A*) negative tests for RV and (*B*) positive tests for RV. The presence of high titers of specific IgE to dust mite in combination with RV leads to greatly increased risk for current wheezing. (*From* Soto-Quiros M, Avila L, Platts-Mills TA, et al. High titers of IgE antibody to dust mite allergen and risk for wheezing among asthmatic children infected with rhinovirus. J Allergy Clin Immunol 2012;129(6):1504; with permission.)

(*P*<.001), arguing that, in the presence of sufficient allergic sensitivity to the dust mite, an RV infection virtually ensured development of an asthma exacerbation sufficiently severe to require urgent care.

The findings of potential synergy between RV infection, allergic sensitization, and asthma exacerbations were further confirmed in controlled trials using omalizumab (anti-IgE) to treat severe or moderately severe asthma.[25,26] Omalizumab used to treat

Table 1
Odds ratio for wheezing based on positive tests for rhinovirus and titers of immunoglobulin E antibodies to dust mite (*Dermatophagoides pteronyssinus*)

Titer of IgE Antibodies to Mite	n	<0.35 IU/mL		0.35–17.4 IU/mL		≥17.5 IU/mL	
		PCR−	PCR+ (A/C)[a]	PCR−	PCR+ (A/C)[a]	PCR−	PCR+ (A/C)[a]
Current wheeze	95	5	4[b] (2/2)	8	16 (3/10)	20	42 (8/30)
Stable asthma	63	12	2 (0/1)	12	5 (1/2)	31	1 (0/1)
Control	123	60	13 (6/4)	31	2 (1/1)	14	2 (1/1)
Nonwheezing children[c]	186	73	15 (6/5)	43	7 (2/3)	45	3 (1/2)
Odds Ratio[d]	—	3.89 (0.9–16), *P* = .07		12.3 (3.8–39), *P*<.001		31.5 (8.3–108), *P*<.001	

[a] Number in brackets indicates the number of subjects positive for group A and group C strains of RV.
[b] Two of these 4 children had IgE antibody to *B tropicalis*: (24.3 and 1.66 IU/mL).
[c] Stable asthma combined with nonasthmatic controls.
[d] Odds ratio for wheezing among RV-positive (real-time PCR) compared with RV-negative subjects.
Adapted from Soto-Quiros M, Avila L, Platts-Mills TA, et al. High titers of IgE antibody to dust mite allergen and risk for wheezing among asthmatic children infected with rhinovirus. J Allergy Clin Immunol 2012;129(6):1503; with permission.

inner-city children had a striking effect in preventing the increase in acute episodes of asthma that occurred in May and September. As previously noted, those months coincide with the season for which allergen exposure is highest and viral infections are prevalent. As also mentioned earlier, during experimental RV challenge, patients with higher IgE levels (>371 IU/mL) have significant changes in bronchial hyperreactivity as judged by methacholine testing and increased symptom severity. Together, these observations strongly suggest that omalizumab likely has a role in mitigating RV-induced exacerbations of asthma. However, controlled trials of anti-IgE treatment before RV challenge, which are ongoing (ClinicalTrials.gov: NCT02388997) will be needed to understand the exact interaction between IgE-mediated allergy and RV-induced exacerbations.

MECHANISMS OF RHINOVIRUS-INDUCED EXACERBATIONS OF ASTHMA RELATED TO ALLERGY

Current research suggests a differential response in asthmatics that consists of cytokines that could bias an allergic response, including interleukin (IL)-25, thymic stromal lymphopoietin (TSLP), and IL-33. In one study, mice that were sensitized to ovalbumin before experimental RV-1B infection showed significantly increased IL-25 messenger RNA (mRNA) levels (28-fold higher than noninfected, allergen-sensitized mice at 10 hours postinfection).[27] Higher IL-25 mRNA levels were associated with increased levels of the T2 cytokines IL-4 and IL-13 in bronchoalveolar lavage fluid 10 hours postinfection and IL-5 at 24 hours postinfection. Moreover, when this group of mice was treated with a monoclonal antibody to block the IL-25 receptor, levels of IL-4, IL-5, and IL-13 decreased and were similar to controls. The researchers from this study corroborated a similar role for IL-25 in human asthmatics, showing that when 28 asthmatics and 11 controls were experimentally infected with RV-A16, asthmatics showed significantly increased levels of IL-25 compared with the baseline before infection.

In the studies mentioned earlier using human PCLS, a role for IL-25 and TSLP was suggested in the increased AHR afforded to human airways after RV infection.[16] In asthmatic tissue, not only was gene expression of IL-25, TSLP, and IL-13 significantly increased at 10, 24, and 48 hours postinfection but TSLP protein release was also significantly increased at 48 hours postinfection (**Fig. 1**B–G). In other studies, TSLP has been induced by both RV infection and double-stranded RNA in the lungs of allergic mice[28] and in human bronchial epithelial cells.[29] Further, TSLP is increased in the nasal passages of young children with RV infection.[30] These findings provide supporting evidence that epithelial generation of T2 cytokines (such as IL-13) leads to increased AHR in the setting of RV infection.

IL-33 has a vital role in the induction and effector phases of type 2 immune responses, and, as such, it is important in many allergic diseases, including asthma, atopic dermatitis, and allergic rhinitis.[31] Genetic polymorphisms of both the IL-33 gene and its receptor are strongly linked to asthma, suggesting atopic individuals may be genetically predisposed to secrete more and respond better to IL-33, especially during allergen challenge.[32] In a recent study by Jackson and colleagues,[33] experimental RV inoculation and bronchoalveolar lavage sampling of human subjects revealed induction of IL-4, IL-5, IL-13, and IL-33 in the airways of asthmatics. Peripheral blood T and ILC2 cells from the same subjects cultured with the supernatants of RV-infected bronchial epithelial cells also induced these cytokines, and this process was entirely dependent on IL-33.[34,35]

FUTURE THERAPEUTIC OPTIONS FOR PATIENTS WITH VIRAL-INDUCED EXACERBATIONS OF ASTHMA

Given the studies that show a muted allergic response in asthmatic patients treated with biologics directed against IgE, it is reasonable to expect lower severity of viral-induced exacerbations because of the lesser T2-biasing response. One such biologic, omalizumab, effectively blocks the activity of much of the circulating IgE by targeting its binding to the high-affinity receptor-binding site on IgE. As a result, omalizumab therapy improves asthma impairment, risk, and degree of control, as shown by reduction in days with asthma symptoms, reduction in exacerbations and hospitalizations, and reduced need for ICS to maintain control.[26] More importantly, as previously noted, the seasonal peaks of asthma exacerbations seen in spring and fall were nearly eliminated in the omalizumab treatment group compared with the control. This association remained in spite of similar detection of viruses throughout the year in both the treatment and control groups.[26] However, because the treatment group reported a significantly decreased number of exacerbations, this further supports the previously discussed synergistic association between viral infections and allergen responses during asthma exacerbations.

In addition to biologics directed against IgE, additional pharmacologic agents have also been developed. Given the central importance of TSLP to RV-mediated asthma exacerbations, it is reasonable to speculate that this agent would also attenuate the presence and severity of exacerbations. A monoclonal antibody to TSLP (tezepelumab) has been evaluated in both an allergen challenge model[35] and in severe uncontrolled asthmatics and was shown to significantly improve asthma control and prevent exacerbations while decreasing eosinophil and exhaled nitric oxide levels.[36] Human monoclonal antibodies to IL-25 and IL-33 are currently also being developed as asthma therapeutics, and the central importance of these cytokines to RV-mediated exacerbations in preclinical studies supports their potential to improve symptoms during RV infections. For example, as previously discussed, blockade of the IL-25 receptor in murine models correlated with decreased T2 biasing response during RV infections.[27] Similarly, in an in vitro study using human asthma bronchial epithelial cells experimentally infected with RV-A16, antibodies to IL-33 resulted in attenuated T2 cytokine production.[33] In summary, these studies support the premise that biologics directed against TSLP, IL-25, and IL-33 could be additional therapeutic targets for prevention of viral-induced asthma exacerbations.

SUMMARY

In recent years, significant progress has been made toward improving asthma control; however, despite these best efforts, there continues to be significant morbidity and, tragically, mortality from asthma. RV is ubiquitous and typically causes only minor upper respiratory symptoms in the general population. However, RV causes asthma exacerbations, especially in the presence of another impetus, especially allergy. Because exacerbations do not happen in every asthmatic with an RV infection, it is possible that exacerbations may be related to the genetic background of the host, occur in the context of a concomitant allergen exposure, or require altered immune responses to the virus that lead to greater inflammation and loss of asthma control. In allergic patients, mechanisms of the host immune response seem to bias toward increased allergic inflammation and worsening AHR. Given these responses, there are several possible treatments available and even more being developed that should improve the ability to control exacerbations related to RV infection.

REFERENCES

1. Mazurek JM, Syamlal G. Prevalence of asthma, asthma attacks, and emergency department visits for asthma among working adults - national health interview survey, 2011-2016. MMWR Morb Mortal Wkly Rep 2018;67:377–86.
2. Zahran HS, Bailey CM, Damon SA, et al. Vital signs: asthma in children - United States, 2001-2016. MMWR Morb Mortal Wkly Rep 2018;67:149–55.
3. Zheng SY, Wang LL, Ren L, et al. Epidemiological analysis and follow-up of human rhinovirus infection in children with asthma exacerbation. J Med Virol 2018;90:219–28.
4. Heymann PW, Carper HT, Murphy DD, et al. Viral infections in relation to age, atopy, and season of admission among children hospitalized for wheezing. J Allergy Clin Immunol 2004;114:239–47.
5. Lee WM, Lemanske RF Jr, Evans MD, et al. Human rhinovirus species and season of infection determine illness severity. Am J Respir Crit Care Med 2012;186:886–91.
6. Castillo JR, Peters SP, Busse WW. Asthma exacerbations: pathogenesis, prevention, and treatment. J Allergy Clin Immunol Pract 2017;5:918–27.
7. Steinke JW, Borish L. Immune responses in rhinovirus-induced asthma exacerbations. Curr Allergy Asthma Rep 2016;16:78.
8. van Benten I, Koopman L, Niesters B, et al. Predominance of rhinovirus in the nose of symptomatic and asymptomatic infants. Pediatr Allergy Immunol 2003;14:363–70.
9. Wildenbeest JG, van der Schee MP, Hashimoto S, et al. Prevalence of rhinoviruses in young children of an unselected birth cohort from the Netherlands. Clin Microbiol Infect 2016;22:736.e9-15.
10. Halperin SA, Eggleston PA, Beasley P, et al. Exacerbations of asthma in adults during experimental rhinovirus infection. Am Rev Respir Dis 1985;132:976–80.
11. Ritchie AI, Farne HA, Singanayagam A, et al. Pathogenesis of viral infection in exacerbations of airway disease. Ann Am Thorac Soc 2015;12(Suppl 2):S115–32.
12. Corne JM, Marshall C, Smith S, et al. Frequency, severity, and duration of rhinovirus infections in asthmatic and non-asthmatic individuals: a longitudinal cohort study. Lancet 2002;359:831–4.
13. Bizzintino J, Lee WM, Laing IA, et al. Association between human rhinovirus C and severity of acute asthma in children. Eur Respir J 2011;37:1037–42.
14. Zambrano JC, Carper HT, Rakes GP, et al. Experimental rhinovirus challenges in adults with mild asthma: response to infection in relation to IgE. J Allergy Clin Immunol 2003;111:1008–16.
15. Adura PT, Reed E, Macintyre J, et al. Experimental rhinovirus 16 infection in moderate asthmatics on inhaled corticosteroids. Eur Respir J 2014;43:1186–9.
16. Zhu J, Message SD, Qiu Y, et al. Airway inflammation and illness severity in response to experimental rhinovirus infection in asthma. Chest 2014;145:1219–29.
17. Kennedy JL, Koziol-White CJ, Jeffus S, et al. Effects of rhinovirus 39 infection on airway hyperresponsiveness to carbachol in human airways precision cut lung slices. J Allergy Clin Immunol 2018;141:1887–90.e1.
18. Loisel DA, Du G, Ahluwalia TS, et al. Genetic associations with viral respiratory illnesses and asthma control in children. Clin Exp Allergy 2016;46:112–24.
19. Hutchinson K, Kerley CP, Faul J, et al. Vitamin D receptor variants and uncontrolled asthma. Eur Ann Allergy Clin Immunol 2018;50:108–16.

20. Bochkov YA, Watters K, Ashraf S, et al. Cadherin-related family member 3, a childhood asthma susceptibility gene product, mediates rhinovirus C binding and replication. Proc Natl Acad Sci U S A 2015;112:5485–90.

21. Stenberg Hammar K, Niespodziana K, van Hage M, et al. Reduced CDHR3 expression in children wheezing with rhinovirus. Pediatr Allergy Immunol 2018; 29:200–6.

22. Kanazawa J, Masuko H, Yatagai Y, et al. Genetic association of the functional CDHR3 genotype with early-onset adult asthma in Japanese populations. Allergol Int 2017;66:563–7.

23. Ayres JG, Mansur AH. Vocal cord dysfunction and severe asthma: considering the total airway. Am J Respir Crit Care Med 2011;184:2–3.

24. Soto-Quiros M, Avila L, Platts-Mills TA, et al. High titers of IgE antibody to dust mite allergen and risk for wheezing among asthmatic children infected with rhinovirus. J Allergy Clin Immunol 2012;129:1499–505.e5.

25. Milgrom H, Berger W, Nayak A, et al. Treatment of childhood asthma with anti-immunoglobulin E antibody (omalizumab). Pediatrics 2001;108:E36.

26. Busse WW, Morgan WJ, Gergen PJ, et al. Randomized trial of omalizumab (anti-IgE) for asthma in inner-city children. N Engl J Med 2011;364:1005–15.

27. Beale J, Jayaraman A, Jackson DJ, et al. Rhinovirus-induced IL-25 in asthma exacerbation drives type 2 immunity and allergic pulmonary inflammation. Sci Transl Med 2014;6:256ra134.

28. Mahmutovic-Persson I, Akbarshahi H, Bartlett NW, et al. Inhaled dsRNA and rhinovirus evoke neutrophilic exacerbation and lung expression of thymic stromal lymphopoietin in allergic mice with established experimental asthma. Allergy 2014;69:348–58.

29. Kato A, Favoreto S Jr, Avila PC, et al. TLR3- and Th2 cytokine-dependent production of thymic stromal lymphopoietin in human airway epithelial cells. J Immunol 2007;179:1080–7.

30. Perez GF, Pancham K, Huseni S, et al. Rhinovirus infection in young children is associated with elevated airway TSLP levels. Eur Respir J 2014;44:1075–8.

31. Ohno T, Morita H, Arae K, et al. Interleukin-33 in allergy. Allergy 2012;67:1203–14.

32. Moffatt MF, Gut IG, Demenais F, et al. A large-scale, consortium-based genome-wide association study of asthma. N Engl J Med 2010;363:1211–21.

33. Jackson DJ, Makrinioti H, Rana BM, et al. IL-33-dependent type 2 inflammation during rhinovirus-induced asthma exacerbations in vivo. Am J Respir Crit Care Med 2014;190:1373–82.

34. Hammond C, Kurten M, Kennedy JL. Rhinovirus and asthma: a storied history of incompatibility. Curr Allergy Asthma Rep 2015;15:502.

35. Gauvreau GM, O'Byrne PM, Boulet LP, et al. Effects of an anti-TSLP antibody on allergen-induced asthmatic responses. N Engl J Med 2014;370:2102–10.

36. Corren J, Parnes JR, Wang L, et al. Tezepelumab in adults with uncontrolled asthma. N Engl J Med 2017;377:936–46.

Rhinovirus Attributes that Contribute to Asthma Development

Mingyuan Han, PhD[a], Charu Rajput, PhD[a],
Marc B. Hershenson, MD[a,b],*

KEYWORDS

- Asthma • Rhinovirus • Innate lymphoid cells

KEY POINTS

- Human rhinovirus infects lower airway epithelial cells and monocyte/macrophages.
- Early-life rhinovirus infection is strongly associated with asthma development in later life.
- The immune system of immature mice and humans is quantitatively and qualitatively different from mature individuals, because it is skewed toward a type 2 cytokine response.
- Stimulation of type 2 innate lymphoid cells by epithelial-derived innate cytokines (interleukin [IL]-25, IL-33, and thymic stromal lymphopoietin) represents a mechanism for viral-induced asthma development.
- Human rhinovirus infection of immature mice, but not adult mice, induces an asthmalike phenotype that depends on IL-13–expressing type 2 innate lymphoid cells.

HUMAN RHINOVIRUS

Human rhinovirus (HRV) is a common and important respiratory viral infectious agent. Since the first discovery in the 1950s, HRV has been identified as the most common cause of upper respiratory tract infection, leading to benign upper respiratory tract illness.[1–3] Advances in molecular methods of viral detection have enhanced the understanding of the spectrum of HRV illness, and HRV infections are now linked to severe bronchiolitis, community-acquired pneumonia, and exacerbations of chronic pulmonary disease, in particular asthma and chronic obstructive pulmonary disease.[4–8]

Disclosure: This work was supported by National Institutes of Health Grant R01 AI120526.
[a] Department of Pediatrics and Communicable Diseases, University of Michigan Medical School, Medical Sciences Research Building II, 1150 West Medical Center Drive, Ann Arbor, MI, USA; [b] Department of Molecular and Integrative Physiology, University of Michigan Medical School, Medical Sciences Research Building II, 1150 West Medical Center Drive, Ann Arbor, MI, USA
* Corresponding author. Medical Sciences Research Building II, 1150 West Medical Center Drive, Ann Arbor, MI 48109-5688.
E-mail address: mhershen@umich.edu

HRV is a member of the family Picornaviridae, genus Enterovirus, carrying a featured positive-sense, single-stranded RNA genome. Similar to other picornaviruses, HRV has an icosahedral, nonenveloped viral capsid consisting of 4 structural proteins: VP1, VP2, VP3, and the myristoylated VP4.[9,10] More than 100 serotypes of HRV have been obtained from the clinical specimens collected in the 1960s and 1970s.[11] Phylogenetic analysis of the available partial sequences of viral capsid-coding regions and noncoding regions, and a limited number of complete genomes, further divided these serotypes into 2 species: HRV-A and HRV-B.[12] These HRV strains were also classified by their receptor specificity, either intercellular adhesion molecule 1 (ICAM-1) (the major group) or low-density lipoprotein receptor (LDLR) (the minor group).[13,14] More recently, a previously unrecognized species, HRV-C, has been found to be a common cause of respiratory illness in humans,[15] and cadherin-related family receptor (CDHR)-3 serves as a receptor for HRV-C strains.[16] With HRV-C, there are now 167 serotypes of HRV.[17]

Until 2 decades ago, the association between HRV and asthma was largely ignored.[18] However, implementation of molecular viral diagnosis provided strong evidence of HRV infection at the lower respiratory tract and suggested a connection between HRV and asthma exacerbation.[19,20] In addition, wheezing-associated viral respiratory infection, especially infection occurring during early life, is now considered a risk factor for asthma development.

During experimental human infection, HRV infects the epithelium of both upper and lower airway.[19,21,22] HRV causes minimal cytotoxicity and infects a small percentage of epithelial cells.[21,23,24] HRV also disrupts the barrier function of polarized airway epithelial cells.[25] The minimal cytotoxicity and small number of epithelial cells infected following experimental infection also suggest that, although epithelial cells may be the major site of viral replication, immune cells may be in large part responsible for the inflammatory response to viral infection. Besides epithelial cells, several other HRV-permissive cell types have been identified. Initially, monocytes and airway macrophages were thought not to be permissive for HRV replication, although HRV enters these cells.[26] Immunofluorescent staining of lower airway specimens obtained from experimentally infected mice[27] and humans has shown the colocalization of HRV with CD68+/CD11b+ macrophages.[28] In addition, HRV replication has been noted in primary human cord blood–derived mast cells, a mast cell line (HMC-1),[29] a basophilic cell line (KU812),[30] and HRV 9–infected[31] and HRV 16–infected[32] human THP-1–derived macrophages. In addition, a recent study suggests that the presence of airway epithelial cells enhances HRV16 replication in monocytic cells by increasing ICAM-1 expression.[33]

As noted earlier, ICAM-1 and low-density lipoprotein family receptors serve as receptors for major and minor HRV-A and HRV-B subtypes, whereas CDHR3 serves as a receptor for HRV-C strains. Accumulating evidence indicates that infections with RV-C are associated with more severe asthma exacerbations, often requiring hospitalization.[15,34–36] Individuals with CDHR3 C529Y variants (AG and AA genotype) seem to be more susceptible to RV-C infection, because this variant is localized on the airway epithelial cell surface, where it is accessible to viral infection, in contrast with the more common GG genotype, which is localized to the cytoplasm.[16,37,38]

Pattern recognition receptors for double-stranded viral RNA, which is synthesized during replication, may also serve as receptors for HRV. The authors have previously shown that Toll-like receptor (TLR)-3 and melanoma differentiation-associated protein (MDA)-5[39] are required for maximal HRV-A–induced neutrophilic inflammation. In addition, we have found that TLR2 expression on the macrophage is required and sufficient for HRV-induced airway inflammation and cytokine expression, and that HRV replication is dispensable for TLR2-HRV interaction.[40]

In healthy humans, experimental infection with HRV induces multiple cytokines and chemokines, including IL-1α, IL-1β, interferon gamma (IFN-γ) and CXCL10. HRV infection of asthmatic patients features increased expression of Th2-related cytokine and chemokines, including IL-4, IL-5, IL-13, CCL11, and CCL26.[41–45] Thus, the cytokine response to viral infection may change based on the lung cytokine milieu; for example, in immature hosts or those with allergic airways disease who are already predisposed to type 2 immune responses. A recent study showed that, following HRV infection, expression of IFN-γ and IFN-λ is higher in asthmatic subjects compared with healthy controls.[45] Natural colds in asthmatic children are associated with increased detection of IFN-γ and IFN-λ messenger RNA (mRNA) in nasal aspirates and higher protein levels of CXCL-8, CXCL-10, CCL2, CCL-4, CCL-5, CCL-11, CCL-19, and CCL-20.[46]

EARLY-LIFE HUMAN RHINOVIRUS INFECTION AND ASTHMA DEVELOPMENT

Early attention to viral infection and asthma development focused on the role of respiratory syncytial virus (RSV). To summarize, community infections with RSV result in asthma-type symptoms but do not lead to persistent wheeze after 13 years of age.[47,48] With the advent of polymerase chain reaction, attention was soon focused on HRV. Among 81 infants hospitalized for wheezing in Finland, HRV had been identified in one-third of infants and was significantly associated with a diagnosis of asthma 6 years after hospitalization. Asthma was present in 60% of the HRV-positive cases.[49] Moreover, in the Childhood Origins of Asthma (COAST) birth cohort, wheezing illness caused by HRV during the first year of life were more strongly associated with persistent wheezing at age 3 years than allergen sensitization or RSV.[50] Nearly 90% of these children who wheezed at age 3 years had asthma at 6 years of age.[51] Furthermore, wheezing with RV, but not RSV, was associated with asthma at age 13 years.[48] Studies from this COAST cohort showed that allergic sensitization precedes HRV wheezing more frequently than the converse, suggesting that wheezing-associated viral infections are not the only factor.[52] Genetic susceptibility at the 17q21 locus is another determinant that has been associated with HRV-induced wheezing illnesses in early life.[53] These clinical investigations not only contribute to the association between early-life HRV infection and asthma development but raise important questions (**Fig. 1**). Does wheezing with HRV infection simply identify children who are already destined to develop asthma? Or could HRV infection in early life, in combination with other factors (allergen sensitization, genetics, or microbiome) lead to the development of asthma?

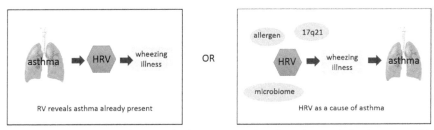

Fig. 1. The potential significance of wheezing-associated respiratory infections caused by HRV, either unmasking preexisting asthma (*left*) or participating in the development of the disease in concert with genetics, environmental exposures, and the microbiome (*right*).

IMMUNE SYSTEM IN ASTHMA
Epithelial-Derived Innate Cytokines

Allergic asthma is associated with eosinophilic inflammation in the lung, enhanced activation of type 2 T-helper (Th2) cells, and excessive type 2 cytokine production, such as IL-4, IL-5, and IL-13.[54,55] The inception of allergic asthma is thought to be associated with sensitization of the airway to common aeroallergens or respiratory pathogens. After sensing the invading foreign substances, immune cells from innate and adaptive immune systems act together with epithelial cells to initiate asthma. Dendritic cells are necessary and sufficient to induce Th2 adaptive immunity to inhaled allergen by presenting the recognized allergen to T cells in the lung lymph nodes.[56] In addition, on allergen stimulation, airway epithelial cells secrete the innate cytokines IL-25 (or IL-17E),[57,58] IL-33,[59] and thymic stromal lymphopoietin (TSLP).[60–63] IL-25, IL-33, and TSLP activate dendritic cells and promote the maturation of Th2 cells.

IL-25 belongs to the IL-17 family and functions as a potent inducer of type 2 immunity.[64] IL-33 is a member of the IL-1 family, which also includes IL-1α/β, IL-18, and IL-1 receptor antagonist. Clinically, adult patients with severe asthma have increased expression of IL-33 in the airway epithelium, endothelium, and smooth muscle.[65] Of note, childhood asthma and wheezing syndromes have been associated with genetic variation in the genes encoding IL-33 and its receptor.[66–68] Moreover, IL-33 expression is significantly induced in submucosal inflammatory cells in pediatric patients with steroid-resistant asthma.[69] Overexpression of TSLP, an IL-7–like cytokine, has been found in the asthmatic airways and is correlated with asthma severity.[70,71] Genome-wide association studies of North American and Japanese populations have found that the TSLP gene locus is associated with asthma risk.[72,73] In addition, several single nucleotide polymorphisms of the TSLP gene locus are associated with asthma development.[74–76]

Although the role of epithelial-derived innate cytokines in allergic asthma is important, these cytokines may also activate type 2 cytokine responses in the absence of allergen or Th2 cells, through their influence on type 2 innate lymphoid cells (ILC2s, discussed later). Moreover, in patients with asthma, experimental HRV infection induces airway IL-33 production that is proportional to exacerbation severity and viral load.[77] HRV infection is associated with increased TSLP levels in the nasal airway secretions of young children.[78] Together, these studies provide a mechanism by which viral infection could induce type 2 airway inflammation and asthma in the absence of allergen exposure.

Type 2 Innate Lymphoid Cell, the Innate Type 2 Immune Effector

The recent recognition of a new innate type 2 immune effector cell, the ILC2, is a milestone breakthrough in allergic disease. ILC is the collective term of a group of hematopoietic cells with a lymphoid morphology that lack rearranged antigen-specific receptors as expressed by T and B cells.[79] Cytokine-producing ILCs are the innate counterparts of the T-helper cell subsets, which function independently of adaptive immunity. ILCs are characterized by the expression of IL-7Rα (CD127) and are divided into 3 groups, group 1 (ILC1), group 2 (ILC2), and group 3 (ILC3), based on their expression of transcription factors and cytokines. ILC2s are considered to be the innate counterparts of Th2 cells based on their expression of transcription factor GATA-3 and production of Th2 cytokines. Similar to Th2 cells, epithelial-derived cytokines IL-25,[80–84] IL-33,[80–82,85–87] and TSLP[87] are essential for ILC2 activation and IL-13 production. ILC2s are considered to be tissue-resident cells that develop early in life.[88] In the lung of newborn mice, ILC2s are almost undetectable.[89] However, the number of lung ILC2s gradually increases, reaching the adult levels around 7 days of life.[90] Compared with adult ILC2s, purified neonatal lung ILC2s produce more IL-5 and IL-13 in vitro.[90] In addition, ILC2s generated in the neonatal period are long lived and persist in adult tissues. Lung ILC2s labeled by bromodeoxyuridine in neonatal mice can be detected in adult lungs.[89]

In contrast with the protective function of ILC2s against allergens and helminths, extensive studies have suggested that dysregulated ILC2 responses contribute to inflammatory processes such as allergic asthma. Analysis of the peripheral blood specimens revealed increased numbers of circulating ILC2s with a greater capacity to produce IL-5 and IL-13[91] and greater pro–type 2 transcriptome expression in the subjects with asthma.[92] In addition, significantly greater numbers of total and type 2 cytokine–producing ILC2s were detected in blood and sputum of patients with severe asthma compared with mild asthmatics.[93] Increased TSLP levels confer steroid resistance on ILC2s from the bronchoalveolar lavage (BAL) fluid of asthmatic patients.[94] In patients with mild asthma, allergen exposure increases the sputum absolute number of ILC2s 24 hours after allergen challenge, paralleling the increased number of ILC2s expressing IL-5, IL-13, or IL-5/IL-13.[91] A recent study showed that ILC2s disrupt bronchial epithelial barrier integrity by targeting tight junctions through IL-13 in asthmatic patients.[95]

RHINOVIRUS–INDUCED TYPE 2 INNATE LYMPHOID CELLS AND ASTHMA DEVELOPMENT IN EARLY LIFE

T-helper 2–Skewed Immune Response in Neonates

Most asthma begins in childhood in association with airways sensitization with aeroallergens and respiratory viral infections. The presence of early-life HRV infection is strongly associated with asthma development. By what mechanism could early-life rhinovirus infection induce development of an asthmalike phenotype?

The immature immune system is qualitatively different from the adult immune system, refractory to type 1 responses, and permissive to type 2 responses.[96–99] In comparison with adult cells, fetal thymic-derived CD4+ T cells showed a Th2-skewed response to antigen.[97] Unlike mature T cells, human cord blood T cells and murine neonatal CD4+ T cells carry a permissive chromatin architecture at CNS-1, a highly conserved, coordinate regulatory region of Th2 cytokine expression.[100,101] Secretion of IL-12 is suppressed in neonatal dendritic cells, thereby inhibiting Th1 cell differentiation.[102,103] With antigen challenge, neonatal basophils secrete IL-4, which binds to the IL-4 heteroreceptor on dendritic cells and reduces IL-12 expression and Th1 cell differentiation in mice.[104] In addition, the type 1 response to TLR ligands is significantly attenuated in neonatal monocytes.[105,106] Thus, type 2–biased neonatal adaptive and innate immune responses could offer a favorable environment for asthma development.

Involvement of Type 2 Innate Lymphoid Cells in Early-Life Rhinovirus Infection

Because early-life viral respiratory infection is associated with asthma, an experimental animal model is essential to elucidate the mechanistic basis underlying viral-induced asthma. In particular, it is of interest to unveil the question of how a chronic disease develops long after the inception of the acute viral infection. Studies have used a mouse model to study HRV-induced disease and exacerbation of allergic airway inflammation.[107,108] The HRV minor group receptors of the LDLR superfamily are evolutionarily highly conserved throughout species, and minor group HRV serotypes infect mouse cells in vitro.[109,110] Thus, infection of mice with the minor group

HRV-1B serotype is localized to the lung and induces strong airway inflammation, albeit accompanied by low viral replication.[107,108] In house dust mite–sensitized adult mice, HRV infection induced exacerbation of allergic airway inflammation and type 2 immune responses.[111]

To evaluate the effects of HRV infection on immature mice, the authors established a model using 6-day-old mice.[112] A delayed and prolonged response to HRV infection was observed that featured increased IL-13 expression, eosinophilic inflammation, mucous metaplasia, and airways hyperresponsiveness.[112] However, HRV infection of mature mice failed to induce eosinophils, mucous metaplasia, or long-lasting airways responsiveness as it did in immature mice. Viral load peaked 3 days after infection of immature mice and, as with adults, decreased progressively thereafter, suggesting that the age-dependent effect was not caused by increased susceptibility of immature mice. Instead, we hypothesized that the immature immune response against HRV infection predisposes baby mice to asthma development.

Compared with adult mice, infection of 6-day-old mice with HRV shows an enhanced type 2 immune response with increased IL-4, IL-5, and IL-13 but attenuated type 1 IFN-γ and IL-12 responses.[113] Studies in progressively more mature mice show that this pattern of type 2 responses switches to the mature type 1 response at approximately 10 days of age. Importantly, a developmental difference in the IL-25 response to HRV infection is also observed. Epithelial-derived IL-25 is increased in HRV-infected immature mice but not in adult mice, which in turn is associated with an increase in the population of IL-25–responsive ILC2s in the immature lung.[113]

Subsequently, it was shown that mature ILC2s are ST2+/TSLPR+ (thymic stromal lymphopoietin receptor [TSLPR]) but express low level of IL-25 receptor (IL-25R), and as a result intranasal administration of IL-25 did not activate lung ILC2s in naive mice.[114] However, expression of IL17-RB, a subunit of IL-25 receptor, was increased in HRV-induced ILC2s.[113] Furthermore, lung ILC2s from HRV-infected mice were required and sufficient for development of the asthmalike phenotype in immature mice. Giving SR3335, a chemical inhibitor of RAR-related orphan receptor alpha (RORα), decreased the number of lung ILC2s and lung mRNA expression of *Il13*, *Muc5ac*, and *Gob5*, as well as mucous metaplasia.[115] In addition, adoptive transfer of ILC2s led to development of an asthmalike phenotype in both immature and adult mice,[115] suggesting the indispensability of ILC2 in the early-life infection of HRV.

We also examined the interrelated effects of the 3 epithelial-derived innate cytokines in our model. Neutralizing antibody against IL-25 abolished HRV-induced ILC2 expansion, mucous metaplasia, and airways hyperresponsiveness. Moreover, increased lung IL-33 and TSLP levels were observed in HRV-infected immature mice, and anti–IL-33 treatment and TSLPR deficiency each significantly attenuated HRV-induced ILC2 expansion and the asthmalike phenotype.[116] IL-33 and TSLP were required for RV-induced IL-25 expression and deposition in the airway epithelium, whereas IL-33 and TSLP had no effect on each other. In addition, TSLP, IL-25, and IL-33 had additive effects on ILC2 function by augmenting cellular responsiveness to each other via upregulation of their cellular receptors.[116]

OTHER FACTORS CONTRIBUTING TO HUMAN RHINOVIRUS–INDUCED ASTHMA

Epithelial-derived innate cytokines IL-25, IL-33, and TSLP, and ILC2-secreted Th2 cytokines, IL-5, and IL-13, are essential for HRV-induced asthma development in immature mice. In addition to ILC2s in immature mice, CD11b+/M2-polarized exudative macrophages are also a cellular source of IL-13 in response to HRV infection of allergen-treated adult mice.[117] Little is known about whether CD11b+/M2 macrophages produce IL-13 during HRV infection of immature mice. Moreover, basophils and mast cells also produce IL-13.[118,119] In HRV-permissive cell lines, HRV infection in combination with phorbol 12-myristate 13-acetate (PMA) or immunoglobulin (Ig) E induces cytokine expression of IL-4 and IL-6 in basophils and IL-8 and granulocyte-macrophage colony-stimulating factor in mast cells.[29] In addition, after viral infection of mice with allergic airways disease, IL-25–driven plasmacytoid dendritic cells boost Th2-mediated effector responses.[120]

As noted earlier, it is conceivable that changes in the microbiome could promote viral-induced asthma. Day care attendance, siblings, and virus-associated acute respiratory infections are marked by appearance of respiratory tract *Streptococcus*, *Moraxella*, and *Haemophilus* species,[121] each of which have been shown to increase the risk of asthma development.[122] Detection of these pathogenic bacteria during HRV infection in older children has been associated with increased severity of ensuing respiratory tract illness, including asthma exacerbations.[123]

Much recent work has been devoted toward understanding how certain asthmatic patients may be more susceptible to HRV infection. As noted earlier, individuals with *CDHR3* C529Y variants (AG and AA genotype) seem to be more susceptible to RV-C infection.[16,37,38] In addition, the *TLR2* −16934 polymorphism has been associated with wheeze and bronchial hyperresponsiveness in day care attendees,[124] consistent with the notion that TLR2 expression heightens the inflammatory response to RV and other respiratory viral infections. Another genetic mechanism underlying childhood asthma relates to variants in the 17q21 locus. The 17q21 variants have been associated with HRV wheezing illnesses in early life[53,66,125] and two 17q21-localized genes, orosomucoid-like 3 (*ORMDL3*) and gasdermin B (*GSDMB*) are significantly increased in HRV-stimulated PBMCs.[53] In the lung, *ORMDL3* gene expression is inducible by allergen and Th2 cytokines and is signal transducer and activator of transcription 6 (STAT-6) dependent.[126] Transgenic expression of human ORMDL3 in adult mice reduces HRV viral load as well as HRV-induced airway inflammation.[127]

In addition, higher circulating levels of IgE may suppress the interferon response to HRV, resulting in greater degrees of airway inflammation and potential for airway remodeling and loss of lung function over time.[128,129] The notion that asthmatics have a deficient immune response to HRV and other viruses has not been settled. During experimental colds, asthmatics with strong IFN-γ responses showed milder cold symptoms and more rapid viral clearance.[130,131] Also following experimental HRV infection, viral clearance and airway function correlate with blood and bronchoalveolar (BAL) CD4 cell IFN-γ production.[43] Epithelial and BAL cells from asthmatics show reduced type I and type III interferon responses to HRV infection ex vivo.[132,133] In contrast, 3 groups have failed to show reduced IFN responses in cultured airway epithelial cells from subjects with asthma.[134–136] A recent evaluation of nasal and bronchial cytokines following experimental HRV infection in allergic asthmatics showed higher nasal lining fluid levels IFN-γ and IFN-λ compared with healthy nonatopic controls.[45] Perhaps most importantly, a difference in viral copy number or titer between controls and asthmatics has not been shown following experimental HRV infection.[137]

SUMMARY

HRV is the most common respiratory infectious agent and most common trigger of asthma exacerbations in children. Including the newly discovered species RV-C, there are now 167 serotypes of HRV. HRV uses the cell surface receptors ICAM-1, LDLR, and CDHR3, and viral double-stranded RNA may elicit inflammatory responses via the pattern recognition receptors TLR3, MDA5, and TLR2. During experimental human infection, HRV infects upper and lower airway epithelial cells as well as monocytes and macrophages. In addition to asthma exacerbations, early-life wheezing-associated infection with HRV has been associated with asthma development. The immune system of neonatal lungs is functionally immature, and the imbalance of Th1/Th2 immune responses may predispose HRV-infected neonates to later asthma development. The authors developed an early-life HRV infection model using immature mice to explore the mechanistic basis of chronic asthma development after the acute HRV infection. HRV infection of 6-day-old immature mice, but not adult mice, leads to an asthmalike phenotype featuring mucous metaplasia and airway hyperresponsiveness, which are IL-13 dependent. ILC2s are the major source of IL-13 in response to stimulation by the epithelial-derived innate cytokines IL-25, IL-33, and TSLP. These data provide a mechanism by which HRV infection in early life, in combination with other factors (allergen sensitization, genetics, or microbiome), could lead to asthma development. In humans, certain genetic variants (*CDHR3* C529Y, 17q21, and *TLR2* −16934) may predispose to HRV-induced childhood asthma. Further studies are needed to understand the association between wheezing-associated HRV infections and asthma.

REFERENCES

1. Makela MJ, Puhakka T, Ruuskanen O, et al. Viruses and bacteria in the etiology of the common cold. J Clin Microbiol 1998;36(2):539–42.
2. Arruda E, Pitkaranta A, Witek T, et al. Frequency and natural history of rhinovirus infections in adults during autumn. J Clin Microbiol 1997;35(11):2864–8.
3. Jacobs SE, Lamson DM, St George K, et al. Human rhinoviruses. Clin Microbiol Rev 2013;26(1):135–62.
4. Henquell C, Mirand A, Deusebis AL, et al. Prospective genotyping of human rhinoviruses in children and adults during the winter of 2009-2010. J Clin Virol 2012;53(4):280–4.
5. Xiang Z, Gonzalez R, Xie Z, et al. Human rhinovirus C infections mirror those of human rhinovirus A in children with community-acquired pneumonia. J Clin Virol 2010;49(2):94–9.
6. Garcia-Garcia ML, Calvo C, Pozo F, et al. Spectrum of respiratory viruses in children with community-acquired pneumonia. Pediatr Infect Dis J 2012;31(8): 808–13.
7. Corne JM, Marshall C, Smith S, et al. Frequency, severity, and duration of rhinovirus infections in asthmatic and non-asthmatic individuals: a longitudinal cohort study. Lancet 2002;359(9309):831–4.
8. Greenberg SB, Allen M, Wilson J, et al. Respiratory viral infections in adults with and without chronic obstructive pulmonary disease. Am J Respir Crit Care Med 2000;162(1):167–73.
9. Oliveira MA, Zhao R, Lee WM, et al. The structure of human rhinovirus-16. Structure 1993;1(1):51–68.
10. Hadfield AT, Lee WM, Zhao R, et al. The refined structure of human rhinovirus 16 at 2.15 angstrom resolution: Implications for the viral life cycle. Structure 1997; 5(3):427–41.
11. Conant RM, Hamparian VV. Rhinoviruses: basis for a numbering system. II. Serologic characterization of prototype strains. J Immunol 1968;100(1):114–9.

12. Palmenberg AC, Spiro D, Kuzmickas R, et al. Sequencing and analyses of all known human rhinovirus genomes reveal structure and evolution. Science 2009;324(5923):55–9.
13. Bella J, Kolatkar PR, Marlor CW, et al. The structure of the two amino-terminal domains of human ICAM-1 suggests how it functions as a rhinovirus receptor and as an LFA-1 integrin ligand. Proc Natl Acad Sci U S A 1998;95(8):4140–5.
14. Vlasak M, Roivainen M, Reithmayer M, et al. The minor receptor group of human rhinovirus (HRV) includes HRV23 and HRV25, but the presence of a lysine in the VP1 HI loop is not sufficient for receptor binding. J Virol 2005;79(12):7389–95.
15. Lee W-M, Kiesner C, Pappas T, et al. A diverse group of previously unrecognized human rhinoviruses are common causes of respiratory illnesses in infants. PLoS One 2007;2(10):e966.
16. Bochkov YA, Watters K, Ashraf S, et al. Cadherin-related family member 3, a childhood asthma susceptibility gene product, mediates rhinovirus C binding and replication. Proc Natl Acad Sci U S A 2015;112(17):5485–90.
17. Palmenberg AC, Gern JE. Classification and evolution of human rhinoviruses. In: Jans DA, Ghildyal R, editors. Rhinoviruses: methods and protocols. New York: Springer; 2015. p. 1–10.
18. Halperin SA, Eggleston PA, Hendley JO, et al. Pathogenesis of lower respiratory tract symptoms in experimental rhinovirus infection. Am Rev Respir Dis 1983; 128:806–10.
19. Gern JE, Galagan DM, Jarjour NN, et al. Detection of rhinovirus RNA in lower airway cells during experimentally induced infection. Am J Respir Crit Care Med 1997;155(3):1159–61.
20. Johnston SL. Natural and experimental rhinovirus infections of the lower respiratory tract. Am J Respir Crit Care Med 1995;152(4 Pt 2):S46–52.
21. Arruda E, Boyle TR, Winther B, et al. Localization of human rhinovirus replication in the upper respiratory tract by in situ hybridization. J Infect Dis 1995;171(5):1329–33.
22. Johnston SL, Papi A, Bates PJ, et al. Low grade rhinovirus infection induces a prolonged release of IL-8 in pulmonary epithelium. J Immunol 1998;160(12):6172–81.
23. Winther B, Gwaltney JM, Hendley JO. Respiratory virus infection of monolayer cultures of human nasal epithelial cells. Am Rev Respir Dis 1990;141(4 Pt 1):839–45.
24. Mosser AG, Vrtis R, Burchell L, et al. Quantitative and qualitative analysis of rhinovirus infection in bronchial tissues. Am J Respir Crit Care Med 2005; 171(6):645–51.
25. Sajjan U, Wang Q, Zhao Y, et al. Rhinovirus disrupts the barrier function of polarized airway epithelial cells. Am J Respir Crit Care Med 2008;178(12):1271–81.
26. Gern JE, Galagan DM, Dick EC. Rhinovirus enters but does not replicate inside airway macrophages. J Allergy Clin Immunol 1994;93(1):203.
27. Nagarkar DR, Bowman ER, Schneider D, et al. Rhinovirus infection of allergen-sensitized and -challenged mice induces eotaxin release from functionally polarized macrophages. J Immunol 2010;185:2525–35.
28. Bentley JK, Sajjan US, Dzaman MB, et al. Rhinovirus colocalizes with CD68- and CD11b-positive macrophages following experimental infection in humans. J Allergy Clin Immunol 2013;132(3):758–61.
29. Hosoda M, Yamaya M, Suzuki T, et al. Effects of rhinovirus infection on histamine and cytokine production by cell lines from human mast cells and basophils. J Immunol 2002;169(3):1482–91.

30. Akoto C, Davies DE, Swindle EJ. Mast cells are permissive for rhinovirus replication: potential implications for asthma exacerbations. Clin Exp Allergy 2017; 47(3):351–60.
31. Johnston SL, Papi A, Monick MM, et al. Rhinoviruses induce interleukin-8 mRNA and protein production in human monocytes. J Infect Dis 1997;175(2):323–9.
32. Laza-Stanca V, Stanciu LA, Message SD, et al. Rhinovirus replication in human macrophages induces NF-κB-dependent tumor necrosis factor alpha production. J Virol 2006;80(16):8248–58.
33. Zhou X, Zhu L, Lizarraga R, et al. Human Airway epithelial cells direct significant rhinovirus replication in monocytic cells by enhancing ICAM1 expression. Am J Respir Cell Mol Biol 2017;57(2):216–25.
34. Miller EK, Edwards KM, Weinberg GA, et al. A novel group of rhinoviruses is associated with asthma hospitalizations. J Allergy Clin Immunol 2009;123(1): 98–104.
35. Khetsuriani N, Lu X, Teague WG, et al. Novel human rhinoviruses and exacerbation of asthma in children. Emerg Infect Dis 2008;14(11):1793.
36. Renwick N, Schweiger B, Kapoor V, et al. A recently identified rhinovirus genotype is associated with severe respiratory-tract infection in children in Germany. J Infect Dis 2007;196(12):1754–60.
37. Bønnelykke K, Sleiman P, Nielsen K, et al. A genome-wide association study identifies CDHR3 as a susceptibility locus for early childhood asthma with severe exacerbations. Nat Genet 2013;46:51.
38. Bønnelykke K, Coleman AT, Evans MD, et al. Cadherin-related family member 3 genetics and rhinovirus c respiratory illnesses. Am J Respir Crit Care Med 2018; 197(5):589–94.
39. Wang Q, Miller DJ, Bowman ER, et al. MDA5 and TLR3 initiate pro-inflammatory signaling pathways leading to rhinovirus-induced airways inflammation and hyperresponsiveness. PLoS Pathog 2011;7(5):e1002070.
40. Han M, Chung Y, Hong JY, et al. Toll-like receptor 2-expressing macrophages are required and sufficient for rhinovirus-induced airway inflammation. J Allergy Clin Immunol 2016;138(6):1619–30.
41. Yoon HJ, Zhu Z, Gwaltney JM, et al. Rhinovirus regulation of IL-1 receptor antagonist in vivo and in vitro: A potential mechanism of symptom resolution. J Immunol 1999;162(12):7461–9.
42. Spurrell JC, Wiehler S, Zaheer RS, et al. Human airway epithelial cells produce IP-10 (CXCL10) in vitro and in vivo upon rhinovirus infection. Am J Physiol Lung Cell Mol Physiol 2005;289:L85–95.
43. Message SD, Laza-Stanca V, Mallia P, et al. Rhinovirus-induced lower respiratory illness is increased in asthma and related to virus load and Th1/2 cytokine and IL-10 production. Proc Natl Acad Sci U S A 2008;105(36):13562–7.
44. Adura PT, Reed E, Macintyre J, et al. Experimental rhinovirus 16 infection in moderate asthmatics on inhaled corticosteroids. Eur Respir J 2014;43(4): 1186–9.
45. Hansel TT, Tunstall T, Trujillo-Torralbo M-B, et al. A Comprehensive evaluation of nasal and bronchial cytokines and chemokines following experimental rhinovirus infection in allergic asthma: Increased interferons (IFN-γ and IFN-λ) and type 2 inflammation (IL-5 and IL-13). EBioMedicine 2017;19:128–38.
46. Lewis TC, Henderson TA, Ramirez IA, et al. Nasal cytokine responses to natural colds in asthmatic children. Clin Exp Allergy 2012;42(12):1734–44.
47. Stein RT, Sherrill D, Morgan WJ, et al. Respiratory syncytial virus in early life and risk of wheeze and allergy by age 13 years. Lancet 1999;354(9178):541–5.

48. Rubner FJ, Jackson DJ, Evans MD, et al. Early life rhinovirus wheezing, allergic sensitization, and asthma risk at adolescence. J Allergy Clin Immunol 2017; 139(2):501–7.
49. Kotaniemi-Syrjanen A, Vainionpaa R, Reijonen TM, et al. Rhinovirus-induced wheezing in infancy-the first sign of childhood asthma? J Allergy Clin Immunol 2003;111(1):66–71.
50. Lemanske RF Jr, Jackson DJ, Gangnon RE, et al. Rhinovirus illnesses during infancy predict subsequent childhood wheezing. J Allergy Clin Immunol 2005; 116(3):571–7.
51. Jackson DJ, Gangnon RE, Evans MD, et al. Wheezing rhinovirus illnesses in early life predict asthma development in high-risk children. Am J Respir Crit Care Med 2008;178(7):667–72.
52. Jackson DJ, Evans MD, Gangnon RE, et al. Evidence for a causal relationship between allergic sensitization and rhinovirus wheezing in early life. Am J Respir Crit Care Med 2012;185(3):281–5.
53. Caliskan M, Bochkov YA, Kreiner-Moller E, et al. Rhinovirus wheezing illness and genetic risk of childhood-onset asthma. N Engl J Med 2013;368(15):1398–407.
54. Robinson DS, Hamid Q, Ying S, et al. Predominant Th2-like bronchoalveolar T-lymphocyte population in atopic asthma. N Engl J Med 1992;326(5):298–304.
55. Woodruff PG, Modrek B, Choy DF, et al. T-helper type 2–driven inflammation defines major subphenotypes of asthma. Am J Respir Crit Care Med 2009;180(5): 388–95.
56. Lambrecht BN, Hammad H. Lung dendritic cells in respiratory viral infection and asthma: from protection to immunopathology. Annu Rev Immunol 2012;30: 243–70.
57. Kaiko GE, Phipps S, Angkasekwinai P, et al. NK cell deficiency predisposes to viral-induced Th2-type allergic inflammation via epithelial-derived IL-25. J Immunol 2010;185(8):4681–90.
58. Gregory LG, Mathie SA, Walker SA, et al. Overexpression of Smad2 drives house dust mite-mediated airway remodeling and airway hyperresponsiveness via activin and IL-25. Am J Respir Crit Care Med 2010;182(2):143–54.
59. Rank MA, Kobayashi T, Kozaki H, et al. IL-33-activated dendritic cells induce an atypical Th2-type response. J Allergy Clin Immunol 2009;123(5):1047–54.
60. Soumelis V, Reche PA, Kanzler H, et al. Human epithelial cells trigger dendritic cell-mediated allergic inflammation by producing TSLP. Nat Immunol 2002;3(7): 673–80.
61. Al-Shami A, Spolski R, Kelly J, et al. A role for TSLP in the development of inflammation in an asthma model. J Exp Med 2005;202(6):829–39.
62. Zhou BH, Comeau MR, De Smedt T, et al. Thymic stromal lymphopoietin as a key initiator of allergic airway inflammation in mice. Nat Immunol 2005;6(10): 1047–53.
63. Ito T, Wang Y-H, Duramad O, et al. TSLP-activated dendritic cells induce an inflammatory T helper type 2 cell response through OX40 ligand. J Exp Med 2005; 202(9):1213–23.
64. Fort MM, Cheung J, Yen D, et al. IL-25 induces IL-4, IL-5, and IL-13 and Th2-associated pathologies in vivo. Immunity 2001;15(6):985–95.
65. Préfontaine D, Lajoie-Kadoch S, Foley S, et al. Increased expression of IL-33 in severe asthma: evidence of expression by airway smooth muscle cells. J Immunol 2009;183(8):5094–103.
66. Moffatt MF, Gut IG, Demenais F, et al. A large-scale, consortium-based genome-wide association study of asthma. N Engl J Med 2010;363(13):1211–21.

67. Belpinati F, Malerba G, Trabetti E, et al. Association of childhood allergic asthma with markers flanking the IL33 gene in Italian families. J Allergy Clin Immunol 2011;128(3):667–8.

68. Savenije OE, Mahachie John JM, Granell R, et al. Association of IL33–IL-1 receptor–like 1 (IL1RL1) pathway polymorphisms with wheezing phenotypes and asthma in childhood. J Allergy Clin Immunol 2014;134(1):170–7.

69. Saglani S, Lui S, Ullmann N, et al. IL-33 promotes airway remodeling in pediatric patients with severe steroid-resistant asthma. J Allergy Clin Immunol 2013; 132(3):676–85.

70. Ying S, O'Connor B, Ratoff J, et al. Thymic stromal lymphopoietin expression is increased in asthmatic airways and correlates with expression of Th2-attracting chemokines and disease severity. J Immunol 2005;174(12):8183–90.

71. Ying S, O'Connor B, Ratoff J, et al. Expression and cellular provenance of thymic stromal lymphopoietin and chemokines in patients with severe asthma and chronic obstructive pulmonary disease. J Immunol 2008;181(4):2790–8.

72. Torgerson DG, Ampleford EJ, Chiu GY, et al. Meta-analysis of genome-wide association studies of asthma in ethnically diverse North American populations. Nat Genet 2011;43(9):887–92.

73. Hirota T, Takahashi A, Kubo M, et al. Genome-wide association study identifies three new susceptibility loci for adult asthma in the Japanese population. Nat Genet 2011;43(9):893–6.

74. Harada M, Hirota T, Jodo AI, et al. Thymic stromal lymphopoietin gene promoter polymorphisms are associated with susceptibility to bronchial asthma. Am J Respir Cell Mol Biol 2011;44(6):787–93.

75. Hunninghake GM, Soto-Quirós ME, Avila L, et al. TSLP polymorphisms are associated with asthma in a sex-specific fashion. Allergy 2010;65(12):1566–75.

76. Myers JMB, Martin LJ, Kovacic MB, et al. Epistasis between serine protease inhibitor Kazal-type 5 (SPINK5) and thymic stromal lymphopoietin (TSLP) genes contributes to childhood asthma. J Allergy Clin Immunol 2014;134(4):891–9.

77. Jackson DJ, Makrinioti H, Rana BM, et al. IL-33-dependent type 2 inflammation during rhinovirus-induced asthma exacerbations *in vivo*. Am J Respir Crit Care Med 2014;190(12):1373–82.

78. Perez GF, Pancham K, Huseni S, et al. Rhinovirus infection in young children is associated with elevated airway TSLP levels. Eur Respir J 2014;44(4):1075–8.

79. Spits H, Di Santo JP. The expanding family of innate lymphoid cells: regulators and effectors of immunity and tissue remodeling. Nat Immunol 2011;12(1):21–7.

80. Neill DR, Wong SH, Bellosi A, et al. Nuocytes represent a new innate effector leukocyte that mediates type-2 immunity. Nature 2010;464(7293):1367–70.

81. Price AE, Liang HE, Sullivan BM, et al. Systemically dispersed innate IL-13-expressing cells in type 2 immunity. Proc Natl Acad Sci U S A 2010; 107(25):11489–94.

82. Mjosberg JM, Trifari S, Crellin NK, et al. Human IL-25- and IL-33-responsive type 2 innate lymphoid cells are defined by expression of CRTH2 and CD161. Nat Immunol 2011;12(11):1055–62.

83. Barlow JL, Bellosi A, Hardman CS, et al. Innate IL-13-producing nuocytes arise during allergic lung inflammation and contribute to airways hyperreactivity. J Allergy Clin Immunol 2012;129(1):191–8.

84. Saenz SA, Siracusa MC, Perrigoue JG, et al. IL25 elicits a multipotent progenitor cell population that promotes Th2 cytokine responses. Nature 2010;464(7293): 1362–6.

85. Moro K, Yamada T, Tanabe M, et al. Innate production of Th2 cytokines by adipose tissue-associated c-Kit+Sca-1+ lymphoid cells. Nature 2010;463(7280):540–4.

86. Chang Y-J, Kim HY, Albacker LA, et al. Innate lymphoid cells mediate influenza-induced airway hyper-reactivity independently of adaptive immunity. Nat Immunol 2011;12(7):631–8.

87. Halim TY, Krauss RH, Sun AC, et al. Lung natural helper cells are a critical source of Th2 cell-type cytokines in protease allergen-induced airway inflammation. Immunity 2012;36(3):451–63.

88. Martinez-Gonzalez I, Ghaedi M, Steer CA, et al. ILC2 memory: Recollection of previous activation. Immunol Rev 2018;283(1):41–53.

89. Ghaedi M, Steer CA, Martinez-Gonzalez I, et al. Common-lymphoid-progenitor-independent pathways of innate and T lymphocyte development. Cell Rep 2016;15(3):471–80.

90. Steer CA, Martinez-Gonzalez I, Ghaedi M, et al. Group 2 innate lymphoid cell activation in the neonatal lung drives type 2 immunity and allergen sensitization. J Allergy Clin Immunol 2017;140(2):593–5.

91. Chen R, Smith SG, Salter B, et al. Allergen-induced increases in sputum levels of group 2 innate lymphoid cells in subjects with asthma. Am J Respir Crit Care Med 2017;196(6):700–12.

92. Lombardi V, Beuraud C, Neukirch C, et al. Circulating innate lymphoid cells are differentially regulated in allergic and nonallergic subjects. J Allergy Clin Immunol 2016;138(1):305–8.

93. Smith SG, Chen R, Kjarsgaard M, et al. Increased numbers of activated group 2 innate lymphoid cells in the airways of patients with severe asthma and persistent airway eosinophilia. J Allergy Clin Immunol 2016;137(1):75–86.

94. Liu S, Verma M, Michalec L, et al. Steroid resistance of airway type 2 innate lymphoid cells from patients with severe asthma: the role of thymic stromal lymphopoietin. J Allergy Clin Immunol 2018;141(1):257–68.

95. Sugita K, Steer CA, Martinez-Gonzalez I, et al. Type 2 innate lymphoid cells disrupt bronchial epithelial barrier integrity by targeting tight junctions through IL-13 in asthmatic patients. J Allergy Clin Immunol 2018;141(1):300–10.

96. Garcia AM, Fadel SA, Cao S, et al. T cell immunity in neonates. Immunol Res 2000;22(2–3):177–90.

97. Adkins B. Peripheral CD4+ lymphocytes derived from fetal versus adult thymic precursors differ phenotypically and functionally. J Immunol 2003;171(10):5157–64.

98. Adkins B. Development of neonatal Th1/Th2 function. Int Rev Immunol 2000;19(2–3):157–71.

99. Roux X, Remot A, Petit-Camurdan A, et al. Neonatal lung immune responses show a shift of cytokines and transcription factors toward Th2 and a deficit in conventional and plasmacytoid dendritic cells. Eur J Immunol 2011;41(10):2852–61.

100. Webster RB, Rodriguez Y, Klimecki WT, et al. The human IL-13 locus in neonatal CD4+ T Cells is refractory to the acquisition of a repressive chromatin architecture. J Biol Chem 2007;282(1):700–9.

101. Rose S, Lichtenheld M, Foote MR, et al. Murine neonatal CD4+ cells are poised for rapid Th2 effector-like function. J Immunol 2007;178(5):2667–78.

102. Goriely S, Van Lint C, Dadkhah R, et al. A defect in nucleosome remodeling prevents IL-12(p35) gene transcription in neonatal dendritic cells. J Exp Med 2004;199(7):1011–6.

103. Lee HH, Hoeman CM, Hardaway JC, et al. Delayed maturation of an IL-12-producing dendritic cell subset explains the early Th2 bias in neonatal immunity. J Exp Med 2008;205(10):2269–80.

104. Dhakal M, Miller MM, Zaghouani AA, et al. Neonatal basophils stifle the function of early-life dendritic cells to curtail Th1 immunity in newborn mice. J Immunol 2015;195(2):507–18.

105. Levy O, Zarember KA, Roy RM, et al. Selective impairment of TLR-mediated innate immunity in human newborns: Neonatal blood plasma reduces monocyte TNF-α induction by bacterial lipopeptides, lipopolysaccharide, and imiquimod, but preserves the response to R-848. J Immunol 2004;173(7):4627–34.

106. Sadeghi K, Berger A, Langgartner M, et al. Immaturity of infection control in pre-term and term newborns is associated with impaired toll-like receptor signaling. J Infect Dis 2007;195(2):296–302.

107. Bartlett NW, Walton RP, Edwards MR, et al. Mouse models of rhinovirus-induced disease and exacerbation of allergic airway inflammation. Nat Med 2008;14(2):199–204.

108. Newcomb DC, Sajjan US, Nagarkar DR, et al. Human rhinovirus 1B exposure induces phosphatidylinositol 3-kinase-dependent airway inflammation in mice. Am J Respir Crit Care Med 2008;177(10):1111–21.

109. Reithmayer M, Reischl A, Snyers L, et al. Species-specific receptor recognition by a minor-group human rhinovirus (HRV): HRV serotype 1A distinguishes between the murine and the human low-density lipoprotein receptor. J Virol 2002;76(14):6957–65.

110. Tuthill TJ, Papadopoulos NG, Jourdan P, et al. Mouse respiratory epithelial cells support efficient replication of human rhinovirus. J Gen Virol 2003;84:2829–36.

111. Toussaint M, Jackson DJ, Swieboda D, et al. Host DNA released by NETosis promotes rhinovirus-induced type-2 allergic asthma exacerbation. Nat Med 2017;23(11):1384.

112. Schneider D, Hong JY, Popova AP, et al. Neonatal rhinovirus infection induces mucous metaplasia and airways hyperresponsiveness. J Immunol 2012;188(6):2894–904.

113. Hong JY, Bentley JK, Chung Y, et al. Neonatal rhinovirus induces mucous metaplasia and airways hyperresponsiveness through IL-25 and type 2 innate lymphoid cells. J Allergy Clin Immunol 2014;134(2):429–39.

114. Martinez-Gonzalez I, Matha L, Steer CA, et al. Allergen-experienced group 2 innate lymphoid cells acquire memory-like properties and enhance allergic lung inflammation. Immunity 2016;45(1):198–208.

115. Rajput C, Cui T, Han M, et al. ROR alpha-dependent type 2 innate lymphoid cells are required and sufficient for mucous metaplasia in immature mice. Am J Physiol Lung Cell Mol Physiol 2017;312(6):L983–93.

116. Han M, Rajput C, Hong JY, et al. The innate cytokines IL-25, IL-33, and TSLP cooperate in the induction of type 2 innate lymphoid cell expansion and mucous metaplasia in rhinovirus-infected immature mice. J Immunol 2017;199(4):1308–18.

117. Chung Y, Hong JY, Lei J, et al. Rhinovirus infection induces IL-13 production from CD11b-positive, exudative M2-polarized exudative macrophages. Am J Respir Cell Mol Biol 2015;52(2):205–16.

118. Kroeger KM, Sullivan BM, Locksley RM. IL-18 and IL-33 elicit Th2 cytokines from basophils via a MyD88- and p38α-dependent pathway. J Leukoc Biol 2009;86(4):769–78.

119. Burd PR, Thompson WC, Max EE, et al. Activated mast cells produce interleukin 13. J Exp Med 1995;181:1373–80.

120. Chairakaki A-D, Saridaki M-I, Pyrillou K, et al. Plasmacytoid dendritic cells drive acute asthma exacerbations. J Allergy Clin Immunol 2018;142(2):542–56.
121. Teo SM, Mok D, Pham K, et al. The infant nasopharyngeal microbiome impacts severity of lower respiratory infection and risk of asthma development. Cell Host Microbe 2015;17(5):704–15.
122. Bisgaard H, Hermansen MN, Buchvald F, et al. Childhood asthma after bacterial colonization of the airway in neonates. N Engl J Med 2007;357(15):1487–95.
123. Kloepfer KM, Lee WM, Pappas TE, et al. Detection of pathogenic bacteria during rhinovirus infection is associated with increased respiratory symptoms and asthma exacerbations. J Allergy Clin Immunol 2014;133(5):1301–7.
124. Custovic A, Rothers J, Stern D, et al. Effect of day care attendance on sensitization and atopic wheezing differs by Toll-like receptor 2 genotype in 2 population-based birth cohort studies. J Allergy Clin Immunol 2011;127(2): 390–7.
125. Moffatt MF, Kabesch M, Liang L, et al. Genetic variants regulating ORMDL3 expression contribute to the risk of childhood asthma. Nature 2007;448:470.
126. Miller M, Tam AB, Cho JY, et al. ORMDL3 is an inducible lung epithelial gene regulating metalloproteases, chemokines, OAS, and ATF6. Proc Natl Acad Sci U S A 2012;109(41):16648–53.
127. Song DJ, Miller M, Beppu A, et al. Rhinovirus infection of ORMDL3 transgenic mice is associated with reduced rhinovirus viral load and airway inflammation. J Immunol 2017;199(7):2215–24.
128. Gill MA, Bajwa G, George TA, et al. Counterregulation between the FcεRI pathway and antiviral responses in human plasmacytoid dendritic cells. J Immunol 2010;184(11):5999–6006.
129. Durrani SR, Montville DJ, Pratt AS, et al. Innate immune responses to rhinovirus are reduced by the high-affinity IgE receptor in allergic asthmatic children. J Allergy Clin Immunol 2012;130(2):489–95.
130. Parry DE, Busse WW, Sukow KA, et al. Rhinovirus-induced PBMC responses and outcome of experimental infection in allergic subjects. J Allergy Clin Immunol 2000;105(4):692–8.
131. Gern JE, Vrtis R, Grindle KA, et al. Relationship of upper and lower airway cytokines to outcome of experimental rhinovirus infection. Am J Respir Crit Care Med 2000;162(6):2226–31.
132. Wark PAB, Johnston SL, Bucchieri F, et al. Asthmatic bronchial epithelial cells have a deficient innate immune response to infection with rhinovirus. J Exp Med 2005;201(6):937–47.
133. Contoli M, Message SD, Laza-Stanca V, et al. Role of deficient type III interferon-lambda production in asthma exacerbations. Nat Med 2006;12:1023–6.
134. Lopez-Souza N, Favoreto S, Wong H, et al. *In vitro* susceptibility to rhinovirus infection is greater for bronchial than for nasal airway epithelial cells in human subjects. J Allergy Clin Immunol 2009;123(6):1384–90.
135. Bochkov YA, Hanson KM, Keles S, et al. Rhinovirus-induced modulation of gene expression in bronchial epithelial cells from subjects with asthma. Mucosal Immunol 2009;3(1):69–80.
136. Patel DA, You Y, Huang G, et al. Interferon response and respiratory virus control are preserved in bronchial epithelial cells in asthma. J Allergy Clin Immunol 2014;134(6):1402–12.
137. DeMore JP, Weisshaar EH, Vrtis RF, et al. Similar colds in subjects with allergic asthma and nonatopic subjects after inoculation with rhinovirus-16. J Allergy Clin Immunol 2009;124(2):245–52.

Infant Immune Response to Respiratory Viral Infections

Santtu Heinonen, MD, PhD[a], Rosa Rodriguez-Fernandez, MD, PhD[b,c],
Alejandro Diaz, MD[d,e], Silvia Oliva Rodriguez-Pastor, MD[f,g], Octavio Ramilo, MD[d,e],
Asuncion Mejias, MD, PhD[d,e,g],*

KEYWORDS

• RSV • Rhinovirus • Innate immunity • Adaptive immune response

KEY POINTS

• Infancy represents a critical window when environmental exposures, including viral respiratory infections, may shape the remodeling of the airway and the function of the immune system.
• Innate immune responses evolve during infancy and differ from that of adults, including weaker interferon responses that may explain their increased susceptibility to viral infections.

Continued

INTRODUCTION

Respiratory viral infections represent the leading cause of hospitalization in infants and young children worldwide, and the second cause of infant mortality.[1] Of all

Disclosures: A. Mejias and O. Ramilo have received research grants from Janssen. A. Mejias has received fees for participation in advisory boards from Janssen and lectures from Abbvie. O. Ramilo has received fees for participation in advisory boards from Abbvie, HuMabs, Janssen, Medimmune, Merck, and Regeneron and lectures from Abbvie. R. Rodriguez-Fernandez has received fees from participating in advisory boards and lectures from Abbvie. Those fees were not related to the research described in this article.
 a New Children's Hospital, Pediatric Research Center, University of Helsinki and Helsinki University Hospital, PO Box 347, Helsinki 00029 HUS, Finland; b Department of Pediatrics, Instituto de Investigación Sanitaria Gregorio Marañón (IISGM), Hospital Materno-Infantil Gregorio Marañón, Madrid 28009, Spain; c Section of General Pediatrics, Hospital Gregorio Marañón, Madrid, Spain; d Center for Vaccines and Immunity, The Research Institute at Nationwide Children's Hospital, The Ohio State Collage of Medicine, 700 Children's Drive, Columbus, OH 43205, USA; e Division of Infectious Diseases, Department of Pediatrics, Nationwide Children's Hospital, The Ohio State Collage of Medicine, 700 Children's Drive, Columbus, OH 43205, USA; f Division of Pediatric Emergency Medicine and Critical Care, Hospital Regional Universitario de Malaga, Malaga 29001, Spain; g Department of Pharmacology and Pediatrics, Malaga Medical Shool, Malaga University (UMA), Malaga, Spain
* Corresponding author. Center for Vaccines and Immunity, The Research Institute at Nationwide Children's Hospital, WA4022, 700 Children's Drive, Columbus, OH 43205.
E-mail address: Asuncion.Mejias@nationwidechildrens.org

Immunol Allergy Clin N Am 39 (2019) 361–376
https://doi.org/10.1016/j.iac.2019.03.005
0889-8561/19/© 2019 Elsevier Inc. All rights reserved.

immunology.theclinics.com

Continued

- Young infants lack immunologic memory toward the invading pathogen, and their adaptive immune responses are biased toward tolerance promoting T-regulatory and T-helper 2 immune responses.
- Viral-induced changes in lung remodeling and the immune response during infancy may explain the association between early life respiratory syncytial virus (RSV) and rhinovirus (RV) infections and subsequent development of recurrent wheezing and asthma.

respiratory viruses that affect young children, respiratory syncytial virus (RSV) and rhinovirus (RV) represent the 2 leading pathogens, because of their implications with acute disease and also because of their association with the development of reactive airway disease (RAD)/asthma later in life.[2–4] By 2 years of age, almost all children have been infected with RSV, and almost all infants develop at least 1 RV infection in the first year of life.[5,6] In addition, in a substantial proportion of children who develop asthma, the disease originates early in life with episodes of RSV or RV, especially rhinovirus-C (RV-C)–induced wheezing.[7,8] One possible explanation for why respiratory viral infections early in life might drive RAD, including asthma, is that the antiviral immune response in infants is markedly different from that of adults, and even within the first months of life. In addition, there is increasing evidence of the role of the microbiome in modulating the host infant immune response during the acute disease and long-term respiratory morbidity.[9,10] In this article, the authors review the different components of the infant immune response to both RSV and RV, their differences according to age, and their possible influence in long-term lung morbidity.

THE INNATE IMMUNE RESPONSE

Innate immunity has a key role in orchestrating early responses to RSV and RV infections, providing an early, nonprogrammed first line of defense. The importance of innate immunity is critical in infants, in whom the immune system is still developing and who often lack immunologic memory. Impaired or dysregulated innate immune responses may lead to slow and inadequate viral clearance, enhanced pathology, and greater disease severity during the acute disease, with possible long-term consequences. Furthermore, impaired innate immune responses lead to inadequate adaptive immune responses, poor immunologic memory, and recurrent infections. The different components of the innate immune response to RSV and RV infections are described in this chapter.

Respiratory Epithelium and Pathogen Detection

The respiratory epithelium serves as the target for the infecting virus and has an important role in inhibiting RSV or RV infections. The respiratory epithelium not only acts as a protective barrier that prevents the direct contact between respiratory viruses and airway epithelial cells but also has active anti-inflammatory and immunomodulatory properties, releasing antimicrobial peptides and cytokines that contribute to the recruitment of inflammatory cells.[11]

Respiratory viruses typically infect ciliated airway epithelial cells, with different viruses having variable tropisms to the respiratory tract. Specifically, RSV infects human airway epithelia cells via the apical surface.[12] Different receptors have been identified for RSV-F or RSV-G proteins, in epithelial cells, including toll-like receptor-4 (TLR-4),

CX3chemokine receptor 1 (CX3CR1), annexin, or nucleolin.[13,14] RV also binds to respiratory epithelial cells using receptors that are different depending on the RV species. Rhinovirus-A (RV-A) and rhinovirus-B (RV-B) bind to ICAM-1 and LDLR receptor, whereas RV-C binds to the newly identified CDHR-3 receptor.[15] The attachment of RSV or RV to their receptors elicits an innate immune response that leads to airway inflammation and possibly remodeling. Thus, the airway epithelium along with the resident immune cells, including macrophages, dendritic cells (DCs), and innate lymphoid cells (ILCs), has a critical role in pathogen detection and initiation of the immune response. These cells express pattern recognition receptors (PRRs) that bind to pathogen-associated molecular patterns. Several PRRs are important in recognizing respiratory viruses, including TLR4, TLR3, TLR2/6, TLR7/8, or TLR9, that are expressed on the cell surface, or retinoic acid-inducible gene I (RIG-I) and melanoma differentiation-associated protein 5 (MDA-5), that are soluble PRRs located in the cell cytoplasm.[16] Although the results are contradictory, possibly because of differences in the patient populations studied, single nucleotide polymorphisms in TLR genes have been associated with increased risk and severity to both RSV (ie, TLR-4, TLR-9) and RV (ie, TLR-8) respiratory infections in infants, emphasizing the importance of these receptors.[17,18]

In addition, the nasopharyngeal microbiota seems to modulate both mucosal and systemic host responses to viral infections. In RSV-infected infants, microbiota clusters enriched for *Haemophilus influenzae* and *Pneumococcus* were associated with increased disease severity, enhanced TLR signaling, and overexpression of neutrophil and macrophage pathways.[10]

Interferon Responses

Of all cytokines and chemokines released during RSV or RV infection, interferons (IFNs) are one of the best characterized because of their antiviral properties. It is not surprising that viruses had developed ways to block IFN production, such as the nonstructural (NS1/NS2) RSV proteins that inhibit the production of IFN-α/β.[19] The importance of IFN responses in the defense against respiratory viruses in infants is highlighted by several studies reporting associations between weaker IFN responses, in the mucosal and systemic compartments, and increased disease severity, mostly in RSV-infected infants.[20–23] There are 3 types of IFNs:

1. Type I IFNs (IFN-α/β) have direct antiviral effects, inducing an antiviral state in both infected and uninfected cells through the expression of IFN-induced genes.[24] IFN-α is produced by several cell types, including airway epithelial cells, alveolar macrophages, and monocytes, but at least in RSV infection, plasmacytoid dendritic cells (pDCs) appear to be their primary source. pDCs harvested ex vivo from infants with RSV infection had lower IFN-α production capacity compared with adult pDCs.[25] In addition, a recent study showed that a predominant T helper 2 (Th2), Th17, and type I IFN response in the respiratory mucosa in infants with acute RSV (but not RV) infection was associated with recurrent wheezing during the first 2 years of life.[26] These data emphasize the important differences on immune responses to viral infections according to age and also to the specific virus.

2. Type II IFN (IFN-γ) early on is produced predominantly by natural killer (NK), NK T cells, and type I ILCs. Later, after development of antigen-specific immunity, the main source of IFN-γ is T cells, including CD4$^+$ Th1, and CD8$^+$ cytotoxic T cells. The association between IFN-γ responses and RSV disease severity has been shown in multiple studies. Initial data from studies in animal models and humans suggested that higher IFN-γ responses were directly associated with the

severity of the disease.[27,28] However, a growing body of evidence has shown that the IFN response to RSV is dysregulated. Indeed, infants with more severe disease, (oxygen administration, need for hospitalization, or mechanical ventilation), had lower concentrations of nasal IFN-γ and/or suboptimal expression of blood IFN-related genes, independent of their atopic status.[20–23,29] In children at risk for developing asthma, lower RV-induced IFN-γ responses measured in cord blood samples were associated with recurrent wheezing during the first year of life.[30]

3. Type III IFN (IFN-λ) or mucosal IFNs are structurally and functionally similar to type I IFNs, although bind to a different receptor and control the infection locally rather than systemically. The human airway epithelium mounts virus-specific responses that are likely to determine the subsequent immune responses. Specifically, studies suggest that absence of interleukin-28A/B (IL-28A/B), and IL-29, which belong to the type III IFN family, from epithelial cells after RSV infection, may explain in part the inadequacy of the systemic immunity to the virus.[31] In addition, a recent study showed lower expression of the type III IFN receptor IFNLR1 in respiratory samples from infants less than 6 months of age hospitalized with RSV compared with RV bronchiolitis.[32] Nevertheless, deficient type I (IFN-β) and type III (IFN-λ) IFN responses have been implicated in the increased susceptibility to RV in patients with asthma.[33,34]

Other Cytokines

Other cytokines mediating early local innate immune responses to RSV and RV infections include tumor necrosis factor-α (TNF-α), IL-6, IL-9, IL-10, CXC chemokine ligand 10 (CXCL10; also known as interferon-gamma inducible protein 10 [IP-10]) (IP-10), CXCL8 (IL-8), CC chemokine ligand 2 (CCL2; monocyte chemoattractant protein-1 [MCP-1]), CCL3 (macrophage inflammatory protein [MIP-1α]), or CCL5 (regulated on activation normal T expressed and secreted [RANTES]), among others.[35,36] In addition to their direct cellular effect at the site of infection, these cytokines act as potent chemoattractants, activating and recruiting circulating immune cells, such as neutrophils, NK cells, and cytotoxic T cells, to the airway mucosa.

Until recently, it was postulated that severe RSV infection was associated with an exaggerated inflammatory response. Similar to IFN responses, there is a growing body of evidence suggesting that some components of the host innate immune response are actually inadequately activated or even suppressed in more severe cases.[37–39] Infants with severe RSV infection had lower production of blood TNF-α, IL-6, and CXCL8 after lipopolysaccharide (LPS) stimulation compared with children with milder RSV infection and with age-matched healthy controls.[40] In another study, concentrations of 29 cytokines in nasal wash samples were compared in young infants hospitalized with either RSV or RV bronchiolitis. The study showed that, overall, infants with RSV infection mounted a more robust response and had higher cytokine concentrations than those with RV infection. Nevertheless, concentrations of MCP-1 and IL-1-α in infants with RV, and of platelet-derived growth factor beta [PDGF]-$\beta\beta$), basic fibroblast growth factor (bFGF), and also IFN-γ in those with RSV infection inversely correlated with the clinical disease severity score.[20] In another study, of all cytokines measured in nasopharyngeal aspirates in young infants hospitalized with a first episode of wheezing, only MIP-1α demonstrated a strong and independent association with recurrent wheezing during the first 2 years of life.[41]

Innate Immune Cells

Neutrophils

The most abundant cell type in the airway from infants with RSV and RV bronchiolitis is neutrophils.[42,43] It still remains unclear whether neutrophils have a protective role or if they contribute to the immunopathogenesis of the disease. Neutrophils limit viral replication and spread by eliminating infected cells, but at the same time release enzymes that may damage the surrounding tissues through neutrophil extracellular traps. It is possible that the damage induced by neutrophils during the vulnerable period of lung development in infants with acute RSV or RV infection may play a role in asthma inception having long-lasting consequences.[44] During acute RV infection, both blood and nasal neutrophils increase within the first 72 hours. The high presence of phagocytic cells and proinflammatory mediators involved in granulocyte regulation, such as granulocyte colony stimulating factor and IL-8, correlate with the severity of RV symptoms, even during mild symptomatic illness.[42] In premature and full-term infants with acute RSV infection, neutrophils seem to be the main source of IL-9,[45] a proinflammatory cytokine associated with development of bronchial hyperresponsiveness and asthma.[46]

Eosinophils
The role of eosinophils during RSV infection is still a matter of debate. Original studies suggested that eosinophilic degranulation in infants during RSV infection was associated with airway obstruction.[47] More recently, in vitro studies showed that eosinophils actually facilitated RSV clearance and reduced infectivity.[48] On the other hand, RV infection may induce eosinophil infiltration and activation within the airway, which correlates with changes in airway hyperresponsiveness, especially in patients with asthma.[49] Some eosinophil-released products, such as eosinophil-derived neurotoxin or eosinophilic cationic protein, have antiviral properties, suggesting an innate antiviral role of these cells during RV infection.[49]

Monocytes, Natural Killer, and Dendritic Cells
Alveolar macrophages are thought to have both immunoregulatory and antigen-presenting capabilities during respiratory viral infections. Macrophages can be infected by RSV and RV as demonstrated by ex vivo viral replication in these cells.[50] In peripheral blood, the number of monocytes increases during acute RSV infection regardless of severity. However, in infants with severe RSV infection requiring hospitalization, the proportion of monocytes expressing low levels of HLA-DR is increased, suggesting that monocyte function might be impaired in the most severe forms of the disease.[51]

The numbers of DCs, NK cells, and cytotoxic T cells also increase in the respiratory tract during RSV infection, because they have an important role in controlling viral replication.[52] A decrease in the number and/or function of these cells has been associated with worse clinical outcomes. In fact, lung tissue samples from infants who died with severe RSV infection showed absence of NK cells and CD8[+] T cells, influx of neutrophils and macrophages in lung tissue, and extensive antigen load.[38]

Although pDCs are important producers of type-I IFN (IFN-α), conventional DCs have an important role as antigen-presenting cells, regulating T-cell responses, and activating NK cells. NK cells contribute to early innate immune responses by providing an early source of IFN-γ, activating T cells, and by direct cytotoxic killing of the infected cell.[53] Although the proportion of blood DC or NK cells with an activated phenotype increases during RSV infection, lower DC and NK cell numbers were observed in RSV-infected children versus healthy controls.[39]

ADAPTIVE IMMUNE RESPONSES
Humoral Immune Responses

Infants have decreased antibody responses compared with adults, due in part to their immature/developing immune system with a limited B-cell repertoire and inefficient generation of somatic hypermutations. In addition, the presence of maternal antibodies may interfere with viral-induced immunogenicity.[54,55] These issues are especially challenging for RSV, which typically causes severe disease in infants at a very young age, their first 2 to 3 months of life. On the other hand, RV induce genotype-specific neutralizing antibodies, with little cross-neutralization among the greater than 100 genotypes identified.

Antibody responses to respiratory syncytial virus

In neonates, circulating RSV immunoglobulin G (IgG) antibodies, which are of maternal origin, decrease significantly by ~4 months of age, with an estimated half-life of 30 to 72 days.[56–58] The interference between preexisting maternal antibodies and the infant humoral immune response after acute RSV infection has been shown in studies conducted in different patient populations.[55,59] In addition, antibody responses are possibly influenced by other factors, such as disease severity or age, both associated with impaired IFN responses, that must be activated to promote adequate T- and B-cell immunity.[60] The proof or principle that antibody responses are critical in preventing severe RSV disease has been demonstrated in different randomized clinical trials using monoclonal antibodies (mAb) against the RSV Fusion protein (palivizumab or motavizumab).[61–64] In those studies, the use of mAb as prophylaxis was associated with a significant reduction in hospitalization rates for RSV lower respiratory tract infection (LRTI), indicating that enough concentrations of neutralizing antibodies could be protective. In addition, the prevention of acute RSV disease by either mAb or maternal vaccination in the future may have implications for diminishing long-term pulmonary morbidity.[65] As an example, studies conducted in animal models and the infant population showed a significant decreased in the incidence of subsequent wheezing/RAD in infants who received palivizumab.[66–68]

Antibody responses to rhinovirus

Additional support of the importance of humoral immunity against RV is derived from patients with primary humoral immune deficiency who experience more frequent and severe RV infections.[69] Virus-specific antibodies, both mucosal IgA and serum IgG, increase after 1 week of the acute infection and provide protection from homologous RV infections and disease.[70] It appears that mucosal antibodies have enhanced neutralizing activity compared with systemic antibody responses.[71] The latter also correlates with immunity and with reduced symptom severity.[72]

Cellular Immune Responses

T cells participate in controlling RSV and RV infection through the recognition of viral antigens, facilitating both cytotoxic and antibody-mediated immune responses.

CD8 T-cell responses

After innate immune responses are activated, most of the cells that migrate to the respiratory tract are cytotoxic lymphocytes or CD8$^+$ T cells. Secretion of RANTES and IP-10 (CXCL10) by RV-infected epithelial cells, neutrophils, and phagocytes promote T-cell chemotaxis.[70] CD8$^+$ T cells play a key role in effective viral clearance; in fact, T-cell immunodeficiencies are associated with prolonged viral shedding and therefore with more severe disease and even mortality.[73] In otherwise healthy infants, transient lymphopenia is common and occurs during the first days of RSV or RV infection, when T cells are migrating to the respiratory tract.[74] CD8$^+$ T-cell kinetics inversely correlates with changes in bronchial hyperresponsiveness in the acute infection and reverts to baseline during convalescence, suggesting that T cells contribute to lower respiratory tract symptoms. In addition, it appears that T-cell differentiation into effector memory

RA$^+$ over resident memory T cells (needed for long-term protection) predominates in young infants with RSV or RV infection and is inverted as the infant immune system matures.[75] A recent study showed that symptomatic RV infection in young infants was associated with marked underexpression of adaptive immunity genes, specifically those related to T cells and cytotoxic/NK cell pathways, which was more profound in patients with severe disease.[76] Whether this reflects a failure to mount an adequate response that leads to a more severe illness, or whether it represents a well-controlled early step in the host response that balances the excessive inflammation during the acute viral infection, remains unclear.

CD4 T-cell responses

CD4$^+$ T cells orchestrate the immune response against respiratory viruses. After T-cell receptors are activated, CD4$^+$ T cells differentiate into specific T-helper subsets, including Th1, Th2, Th17, regulatory T cells (Tregs), and T follicular helper (Tfh) cells, which are defined by their function and cytokine milieu (**Fig 1**):

- Th1 cell responses are critical during the acute infection and are mediated mainly by IFN-γ. Other cytokines involved in Th1 immune responses include IL-1, IL-2, IL-12, IL-18, and TNF-α. As discussed previously, impaired type II IFN responses in blood and respiratory samples have been associated with enhanced RSV disease severity.[20,21,73] In addition, although IFN-γ can inhibit IL-4-mediated allergic responses, it may contribute to early wheeze after RV infection (but not RSV) in predisposed infants with atopy.[77]

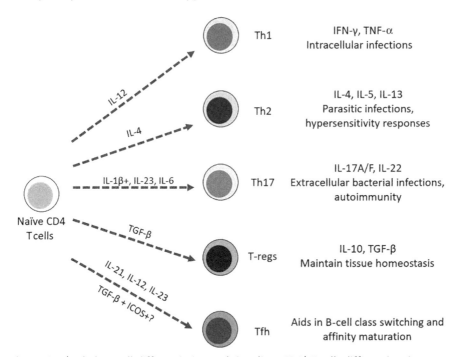

Fig. 1. CD4$^+$ T-helper cell differentiation and signaling. CD4$^+$ T cells differentiate into specific T-helper subsets upon activation of T-cell receptors, including Th1, Th2, Th17, Tregs, and Tfh cells, which are defined by their function and cytokine milieu. ICOS, Inducible T-cell costimulator; TGF-β, transforming growth factor-β.

- Th2 cell responses are defined by the production of IL-4, IL-5, IL-9, and IL-13 and involved in antibody production, class switching, and also eosinophilic responses. Studies suggest that a predominant infant Th2 response during acute RSV infection assessed by decreased IFN-γ/IL-4 ratios is associated with enhanced disease and also development of persistent wheezing.[78–80] There are several factors that could explain persistent wheezing after RSV or RV LRTI, including short- and long-term remodeling of the airway physiology and certainly the airway immune response.

- We are discussing the functions of Th17 cells that include: a) more mucus production, b) enhance Th2 responses, c) modulate CD8 T cells, etc. Th17 cells are defined by the production of IL-17A/F and IL-22, playing an essential role in protection against extracellular pathogens, autoimmunity, and also in the development of some forms of asthma.[81] This third type of CD4$^+$ T cells is considered a bridge between innate and adaptive immunity and has different functions during RSV or RV infections, including favoring an exaggerated mucus production, enhance Th2 responses, stimulate lung neutrophilic infiltration, and modulate CD8$^+$ T-cell responses.[82,83] Higher concentrations of IL-17, but also IL-4 and IFN-γ, were associated with a decreased risk of hospitalization in infants with RSV or RV LRTI, suggesting that there is tremendous overlap on cytokine responses needed to control these virus-induced lung diseases in infants.[29,84]

- Treg cells are responsible for maintaining tissue homeostasis during the acute infection by facilitating viral clearance and avoiding excessive innate (neutrophils/NK cells) and cellular immune responses of both CD4 and CD8 T cells.[82] The main cytokines associated with Tregs are IL-10 and transforming growth factor-β, which play an important role in the delicate balance between Th1, Th2, and Th17 responses.[85,86] IL-10 has important regulatory functions during acute and convalescent RSV and RV infection in infants. Some studies showed the association between increased concentrations of serum IL-10 and acute RSV or RV severity, as assessed by the need for supplemental O$_2$ or viral-induced wheeze, whereas others have shown a protective effect of mucosal IL-10 in regards to hypoxemia and severity.[73] Although IL-12 favors the differentiation of CD4$^+$ T cells into a Th1 phenotype, IL-10 inhibits Th1 responses, thus favoring a Th2 phenotype and development of subsequent wheezing.[87] Moreover, increased serum monocyte-derived IL-10 responses 1 month after acute RSV infection were associated with recurrent wheezing in the first year of life, emphasizing the important regulatory role of this cytokine.[80]

- Tfh cells, recently identified as CD4 T cells, are characterized by the expression of CXCR5 (chemokine receptor), BCL6 (transcription factor), and PD-1 (inhibitory molecule). Tfh cells help with B-cell class switching and are essential for affinity maturation and the development of memory B cells.[88] There is limited information about their role during RSV or RV infection. A recent study in infants with bronchiolitis showed that activation of BCL6 pathways in blood or nasopharyngeal samples was associated with RSV, but not RV, severity.[89]

AGE-SPECIFIC DIFFERENCES IN IMMUNE RESPONSES

The immune cell milieu in infants is immature and changes drastically in their composition and function after birth, especially during the first months of life.[90] The infant's immune response is geared toward Treg and CD4$^+$ Th2 over Th1 responses. This balance may be beneficial in the development of tolerance to self and other antigens, but it may also increase the susceptibility to viral infections.[91] In addition, infants lack immunologic memory toward the invading pathogen, and maternal antibodies provide protection during the first months of life, but the protection is incomplete, especially against mucosal infections, and wanes after 4 to 6 months of age.

Environmental exposures seem to be key drivers in the development of the infant immune response. Thus, infancy represents a critical window that may shape the remodeling of the airway and the long-term function of the immune system, offering a potential explanation for the association between early-life RSV and RV infections, and subsequent development of RAD/asthma. Studies have shown that immune responses are quantitatively and qualitatively different in young infants compared with adults. Stimulation assays with different TLR agonists showed that cord blood-derived white blood cells (WBCs) produced equal or greater amounts of Th2 and Th17 cytokines, but had weaker Th1 responses when compared with adult WBCs.[92] In addition, weaker responses to LPS and lower TLR4 expression were observed in cord blood-derived monocytes compared with adult monocytes.[93] Thus, because pathogen detection is critical for the activation of the immune cascade, and because Th1 type responses and also memory are considered fundamental against respiratory viruses, these age-specific differences could explain in part the increased susceptibility to viral respiratory tract infections in infants.

Host Transcriptional Profiling

Host transcriptional profiling has provided valuable insights into immune responses to respiratory viral infections. Different studies have shown that the systemic immune response to RSV or RV respiratory tract infections is characterized by increased expression of neutrophil-related genes and relative decreased expression of IFN, and B- and T-cell-related genes according to severity.[21,89,94] Importantly, the magnitude of those responses was different according to the respiratory virus and were greatly influenced by age and severity. Preliminary studies in healthy young infants (<6 months) showed that IFN and inflammation genes were underexpressed compared with that of older infants, making infants in early life uniquely susceptible to respiratory viral infections. Recently, transcriptional profiling of nasopharyngeal and blood samples from infants with RSV or RV infection showed similar strong innate and IFN responses in both compartments in RSV-infected infants, whereas RV responses were not as strong and differed between nasopharyngeal and blood samples.[89]

A recent study showed that the immune transcriptional profile of infants less than 6 months old versus 6 to 24 months old was significantly different in response to RSV or RV infection, adjusted for disease severity and other demographic characteristics.[21] Overall, the RSV immune profile in the younger age group was contracted and dominated by a greater proportion of underexpressed transcripts compared with older children (6–24 months). Using several analytical strategies, the study showed that despite these infants being equally ill as reflected by their similar clinical disease severity scores, those of younger age displayed significantly less expression of IFN, inflammation and neutrophil transcripts, lack of activation of plasma cell-related genes, and greater underexpression of B-cell-, NK-cell-, and T-cell-related genes (**Fig 2**A).[21] Furthermore, when the pathways activated or suppressed in infants with RV versus RSV LRTI were analyzed, also stratified by age (<6 vs 6–24 months), significant differences in the expression of several immune pathways were identified. Infants with RV infection, independent of age, demonstrated mild activation of immune response-related pathways, with more subtle differences according to age (**Fig 2**B). Although younger RV infants showed less activation of IFN-related genes, there were no differences in the overexpression of neutrophil, monocyte, or inflammation genes. On the other hand, and similar to that from infants with RSV LRTI, adaptive

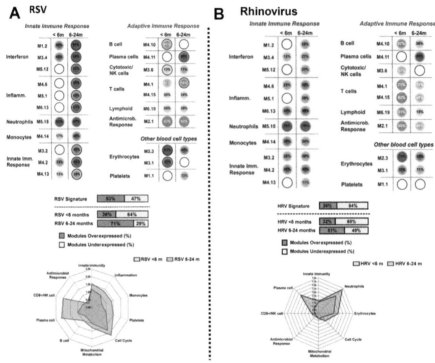

Fig. 2. Age at the time of infection influences the host immune response to RSV and RV infection. (*A*) Immune pathways activated or suppressed during RSV LRTI were compared between 20 infants less than 6 months of age and 17 children with RSV LRTI 6 to 24 months of age (*upper panel*). Both groups had similar clinical disease severity scores. Colored spots represent the percentage of significantly overexpressed (*red*) or underexpressed (*blue*) transcripts within a module, and the number included in the dots is the percentage of overexpressed or underexpressed transcripts. Blank modules demonstrate no significant differences in expression. The middle panel summarizes the percentage of overexpressed and underexpressed transcripts according to the 2 age groups and in relation to the overall RSV signature. The lower panel further illustrates in a spider graph format the differences in immune responses between the 2 age groups. (*B*) Infants with RV LRTI (<6 months, n = 12; and 6–24 months, n = 8) revealed fewer differences in host responses according to age. Horizontal bars illustrate the proportion of overexpressed and underexpressed modules in infants (<6 months) and children 6 to 24 months of age in relation to the global influenza and RV signature. These differences are further illustrated in a spider graph format representing the per-module median expression values of the significant different modules between the 2 age groups. Antimicrob, antimicrobial; HRV, human rhinovirus; Imm, Immune; Inflamm, Inflammation. (*Adapted from* Mejias A, Dimo B, Suarez NM, et al. Whole blood gene expression profiles to assess pathogenesis and disease severity in infants with respiratory syncytial virus infection. PLoS Med 2013;10(11):e1001549; with permission.)

immune response pathways were greatly suppressed in younger versus older children with RV LRTI.[21] These differences in the immune response were observed in symptomatic RV infection versus with asymptomatic RV detection.[76]

These data suggest that although there are pathways that are commonly activated upon infection with different respiratory viruses, the type and breadth of these responses are greatly influenced by age. Nevertheless, whether age at the time of the infection or the observed age-related changes in immune responses influence the subsequent development of asthma or atopy await further study.

SUMMARY

Infancy represents a critical window when environmental exposures, and in particular RSV and RV infections, may shape the remodeling of the airway and the function of a developing immune system. The immune response evolves during infancy and is characterized early on by lack of immunologic memory, and a biased tolerogenic immune response (Tregs and Th2 responses), whereas Th1 immunity is restrained and associated with disease severity. These specific nuances on the immune response may explain the infant susceptibility to these infections and their association with the development of recurrent wheezing/asthma later in life.

REFERENCES

1. Lozano R, Naghavi M, Foreman K, et al. Global and regional mortality from 235 causes of death for 20 age groups in 1990 and 2010: a systematic analysis for the Global Burden of Disease Study 2010. Lancet 2012;380(9859):2095–128.
2. Jackson DJ, Gangnon RE, Evans MD, et al. Wheezing rhinovirus illnesses in early life predict asthma development in high-risk children. Am J Respir Crit Care Med 2008;178(7):667–72.
3. Sigurs N, Aljassim F, Kjellman B, et al. Asthma and allergy patterns over 18 years after severe RSV bronchiolitis in the first year of life. Thorax 2010;65(12):1045–52.
4. Stein RT, Sherrill D, Morgan WJ, et al. Respiratory syncytial virus in early life and risk of wheeze and allergy by age 13 years. Lancet 1999;354(9178):541–5.
5. van der Zalm MM, Wilbrink B, van Ewijk BE, et al. Highly frequent infections with human rhinovirus in healthy young children: a longitudinal cohort study. J Clin Virol 2011;52(4):317–20.
6. Mejias A, Ramilo O. New options in the treatment of respiratory syncytial virus disease. J Infect 2015;71(Suppl 1):S80–7.
7. Miller EK, Bugna J, Libster R, et al. Human rhinoviruses in severe respiratory disease in very low birth weight infants. Pediatrics 2012;129(1):e60–7.
8. Drysdale SB, Alcazar M, Wilson T, et al. Respiratory outcome of prematurely born infants following human rhinovirus A and C infections. Eur J Pediatr 2014;173(7): 913–9.
9. Beigelman A, Bacharier LB. Early-life respiratory infections and asthma development: role in disease pathogenesis and potential targets for disease prevention. Curr Opin Allergy Clin Immunol 2016;16(2):172–8.
10. de Steenhuijsen Piters WA, Heinonen S, Hasrat R, et al. Nasopharyngeal microbiota, host transcriptome, and disease severity in children with respiratory syncytial virus infection. Am J Respir Crit Care Med 2016;194(9):1104–15.
11. Zanin M, Baviskar P, Webster R, et al. The interaction between respiratory pathogens and mucus. Cell Host Microbe 2016;19(2):159–68.
12. Guo-Parke H, Canning P, Douglas I, et al. Relative respiratory syncytial virus cytopathogenesis in upper and lower respiratory tract epithelium. Am J Respir Crit Care Med 2013;188(7):842–51.
13. Johnson SM, McNally BA, Ioannidis I, et al. Respiratory syncytial virus uses CX3CR1 as a receptor on primary human airway epithelial cultures. PLoS Pathog 2015;11(12):e1005318.
14. Tayyari F, Marchant D, Moraes TJ, et al. Identification of nucleolin as a cellular receptor for human respiratory syncytial virus. Nat Med 2011;17(9):1132–5.
15. Bochkov YA, Watters K, Ashraf S, et al. Cadherin-related family member 3, a childhood asthma susceptibility gene product, mediates rhinovirus C binding and replication. Proc Natl Acad Sci U S A 2015;112(17):5485–90.

16. Takeuchi O, Akira S. Innate immunity to virus infection. Immunol Rev 2009;227(1): 75–86.
17. Toivonen L, Vuononvirta J, Mertsola J, et al. Polymorphisms of mannose-binding lectin and toll-like receptors 2, 3, 4, 7 and 8 and the risk of respiratory infections and acute otitis media in children. Pediatr Infect Dis J 2017;36(5):e114–22.
18. Alvarez AE, Marson FAL, Bertuzzo CS, et al. Association between single nucleotide polymorphisms in TLR4, TLR2, TLR9, VDR, NOS2 and CCL5 genes with acute viral bronchiolitis. Gene 2018;645:7–17.
19. Ramaswamy M, Shi L, Monick MM, et al. Specific inhibition of type I interferon signal transduction by respiratory syncytial virus. Am J Respir Cell Mol Biol 2004;30(6):893–900.
20. Garcia C, Soriano-Fallas A, Lozano J, et al. Decreased innate immune cytokine responses correlate with disease severity in children with respiratory syncytial virus and human rhinovirus bronchiolitis. Pediatr Infect Dis J 2012;31(1):86–9.
21. Mejias A, Dimo B, Suarez NM, et al. Whole blood gene expression profiles to assess pathogenesis and disease severity in infants with respiratory syncytial virus infection. PLoS Med 2013;10(11):e1001549.
22. Bont L, Heijnen CJ, Kavelaars A, et al. Local interferon-gamma levels during respiratory syncytial virus lower respiratory tract infection are associated with disease severity. J Infect Dis 2001;184(3):355–8.
23. Piedra FA, Mei M, Avadhanula V, et al. The interdependencies of viral load, the innate immune response, and clinical outcome in children presenting to the emergency department with respiratory syncytial virus-associated bronchiolitis. PLoS One 2017;12(3):e0172953.
24. McNab F, Mayer-Barber K, Sher A, et al. Type I interferons in infectious disease. Nat Rev Immunol 2015;15(2):87–103.
25. Marr N, Wang T-I, Kam SHY, et al. Attenuation of respiratory syncytial virus-induced and RIG-I-dependent type I IFN responses in human neonates and very young children. J Immunol 2014;192(3):948–57.
26. Turi KN, Shankar J, Anderson LJ, et al. Infant viral respiratory infection nasal immune-response patterns and their association with subsequent childhood recurrent wheeze. Am J Respir Crit Care Med 2018;198(8):1064–73.
27. van Schaik SM, Tristram DA, Nagpal IS, et al. Increased production of IFN-gamma and cysteinyl leukotrienes in virus-induced wheezing. J Allergy Clin Immunol 1999;103(4):630–6.
28. Jafri HS, Chavez-Bueno S, Mejias A, et al. Respiratory syncytial virus induces pneumonia, cytokine response, airway obstruction, and chronic inflammatory infiltrates associated with long-term airway hyperresponsiveness in mice. J Infect Dis 2004;189(10):1856–65.
29. Nicholson EG, Schlegel C, Garofalo RP, et al. Robust cytokine and chemokine response in nasopharyngeal secretions: association with decreased severity in children with physician diagnosed bronchiolitis. J Infect Dis 2016;214(4):649–55.
30. Gern JE, Brooks GD, Meyer P, et al. Bidirectional interactions between viral respiratory illnesses and cytokine responses in the first year of life. J Allergy Clin Immunol 2006;117(1):72–8.
31. Ioannidis I, McNally B, Willette M, et al. Plasticity and virus specificity of the airway epithelial cell immune response during respiratory virus infection. J Virol 2012;86(10):5422–36.
32. Pierangeli A, Statzu M, Nenna R, et al. Interferon lambda receptor 1 (IFNL1R) transcript is highly expressed in rhinovirus bronchiolitis and correlates with disease severity. J Clin Virol 2018;102:101–9.

33. Wark PA, Johnston SL, Bucchieri F, et al. Asthmatic bronchial epithelial cells have a deficient innate immune response to infection with rhinovirus. J Exp Med 2005; 201(6):937–47.

34. Contoli M, Message SD, Laza-Stanca V, et al. Role of deficient type III interferon-lambda production in asthma exacerbations. Nat Med 2006;12(9):1023–6.

35. McNamara PS, Flanagan BF, Hart CA, et al. Production of chemokines in the lungs of infants with severe respiratory syncytial virus bronchiolitis. J Infect Dis 2005;191(8):1225–32.

36. Sheeran P, Jafri H, Carubelli C, et al. Elevated cytokine concentrations in the nasopharyngeal and tracheal secretions of children with respiratory syncytial virus disease. Pediatr Infect Dis J 1999;18(2):115–22.

37. Bennett BL, Garofalo RP, Cron SG, et al. Immunopathogenesis of respiratory syncytial virus bronchiolitis. J Infect Dis 2007;195(10):1532–40.

38. Welliver TP, Garofalo RP, Hosakote Y, et al. Severe human lower respiratory tract illness caused by respiratory syncytial virus and influenza virus is characterized by the absence of pulmonary cytotoxic lymphocyte responses. J Infect Dis 2007; 195(8):1126–36.

39. Larranaga CL, Ampuero SL, Luchsinger VF, et al. Impaired immune response in severe human lower tract respiratory infection by respiratory syncytial virus. Pediatr Infect Dis J 2009;28(10):867–73.

40. Mella C, Suarez-Arrabal MC, Lopez S, et al. Innate immune dysfunction is associated with enhanced disease severity in infants with severe respiratory syncytial virus bronchiolitis. J Infect Dis 2013;207(4):564–73.

41. Sugai K, Kimura H, Miyaji Y, et al. MIP-1alpha level in nasopharyngeal aspirates at the first wheezing episode predicts recurrent wheezing. J Allergy Clin Immunol 2016;137(3):774–81.

42. Turner RB, Weingand KW, Yeh CH, et al. Association between interleukin-8 concentration in nasal secretions and severity of symptoms of experimental rhinovirus colds. Clin Infect Dis 1998;26(4):840–6.

43. McNamara PS, Ritson P, Selby A, et al. Bronchoalveolar lavage cellularity in infants with severe respiratory syncytial virus bronchiolitis. Arch Dis Child 2003; 88(10):922–6.

44. Geerdink RJ, Pillay J, Meyaard L, et al. Neutrophils in respiratory syncytial virus infection: a target for asthma prevention. J Allergy Clin Immunol 2015;136(4): 838–47.

45. McNamara PS, Flanagan BF, Baldwin LM, et al. Interleukin 9 production in the lungs of infants with severe respiratory syncytial virus bronchiolitis. Lancet 2004;363(9414):1031–7.

46. Kearley J, Erjefalt JS, Andersson C, et al. IL-9 governs allergen-induced mast cell numbers in the lung and chronic remodeling of the airways. Am J Respir Crit Care Med 2011;183(7):865–75.

47. Garofalo R, Kimpen JL, Welliver RC, et al. Eosinophil degranulation in the respiratory tract during naturally acquired respiratory syncytial virus infection. J Pediatr 1992;120(1):28–32.

48. Rosenberg HF, Dyer KD, Domachowske JB. Eosinophils and their interactions with respiratory virus pathogens. Immunol Res 2009;43(1–3):128–37.

49. Rosenberg HF, Domachowske JB. Eosinophils, eosinophil ribonucleases, and their role in host defense against respiratory virus pathogens. J Leukoc Biol 2001;70(5):691–8.

50. Midulla F, Villani A, Panuska JR, et al. Respiratory syncytial virus lung infection in infants: immunoregulatory role of infected alveolar macrophages. J Infect Dis 1993;168(6):1515–9.

51. Ahout IM, Jans J, Haroutiounian L, et al. Reduced expression of HLA-DR on monocytes during severe respiratory syncytial virus infections. Pediatr Infect Dis J 2016;35(3):e89–96.

52. Gill MA, Palucka AK, Barton T, et al. Mobilization of plasmacytoid and myeloid dendritic cells to mucosal sites in children with respiratory syncytial virus and other viral respiratory infections. J Infect Dis 2005;191(7):1105–15.

53. Culley FJ. Natural killer cells in infection and inflammation of the lung. Immunology 2009;128(2):151–63.

54. Murphy BR, Alling DW, Snyder MH, et al. Effect of age and preexisting antibody on serum antibody response of infants and children to the F and G glycoproteins during respiratory syncytial virus infection. J Clin Microbiol 1986;24(5):894–8.

55. Trento A, Rodriguez-Fernandez R, Gonzalez-Sanchez MI, et al. The complexity of antibody responses elicited against the respiratory syncytial virus glycoproteins in hospitalized children younger than 2 years. Front Microbiol 2017;8:2301.

56. Capella C, Chaiwatpongsakorn S, Gorrell E, et al. Antibodies, and disease severity in infants and young children with acute respiratory syncytial virus infection. J Infect Dis 2017;216(11):1398–406.

57. Chu HY, Steinhoff MC, Magaret A, et al. Respiratory syncytial virus transplacental antibody transfer and kinetics in mother-infant pairs in Bangladesh. J Infect Dis 2014;210(10):1582–9.

58. Ochola R, Sande C, Fegan G, et al. The level and duration of RSV-specific maternal IgG in infants in Kilifi Kenya. PLoS One 2009;4(12):e8088.

59. Shinoff JJ, O'Brien KL, Thumar B, et al. Young infants can develop protective levels of neutralizing antibody after infection with respiratory syncytial virus. J Infect Dis 2008;198(7):1007–15.

60. Swanson CL, Wilson TJ, Strauch P, et al. Type I IFN enhances follicular B cell contribution to the T cell-independent antibody response. J Exp Med 2010; 207(7):1485–500.

61. Palivizumab, a humanized respiratory syncytial virus monoclonal antibody, reduces hospitalization from respiratory syncytial virus infection in high-risk infants. Pediatrics 1998;102(3):531–7.

62. Feltes TF, Cabalka AK, Meissner HC, et al. Palivizumab prophylaxis reduces hospitalization due to respiratory syncytial virus in young children with hemodynamically significant congenital heart disease. J Pediatr 2003;143(4):532–40.

63. Carbonell-Estrany X, Simoes EA, Dagan R, et al. Motavizumab for prophylaxis of respiratory syncytial virus in high-risk children: a noninferiority trial. Pediatrics 2010;125(1):e35–51.

64. O'Brien KL, Chandran A, Weatherholtz R, et al. Efficacy of motavizumab for the prevention of respiratory syncytial virus disease in healthy Native American infants: a phase 3 randomised double-blind placebo-controlled trial. Lancet Infect Dis 2015;15(12):1398–408.

65. Mejias A, Garcia-Maurino C, Rodriguez-Fernandez R, et al. Development and clinical applications of novel antibodies for prevention and treatment of respiratory syncytial virus infection. Vaccine 2017;35(3):496–502.

66. Blanken MO, Rovers MM, Molenaar JM, et al. Respiratory syncytial virus and recurrent wheeze in healthy preterm infants. N Engl J Med 2013;368(19):1791–9.

67. Mejias A, Chavez-Bueno S, Rios AM, et al. Anti-respiratory syncytial virus (RSV) neutralizing antibody decreases lung inflammation, airway obstruction, and

airway hyperresponsiveness in a murine RSV model. Antimicrob Agents Chemother 2004;48(5):1811–22.

68. Mochizuki H, Kusuda S, Okada K, et al. Palivizumab prophylaxis in preterm infants and subsequent recurrent wheezing. Six-year follow-up study. Am J Respir Crit Care Med 2017;196(1):29–38.

69. Kainulainen L, Vuorinen T, Rantakokko-Jalava K, et al. Recurrent and persistent respiratory tract viral infections in patients with primary hypogammaglobulinemia. J Allergy Clin Immunol 2010;126(1):120–6.

70. Jacobs SE, Lamson DM, St George K, et al. Human rhinoviruses. Clin Microbiol Rev 2013;26(1):135–62.

71. Perkins JC, Tucker DN, Knopf HL, et al. Comparison of protective effect of neutralizing antibody in serum and nasal secretions in experimental rhinovirus type 13 illness. Am J Epidemiol 1969;90(6):519–26.

72. Butler WT, Waldmann TA, Rossen RD, et al. Changes in IgA and IgG concentrations in nasal secretions prior to the appearance of antibody during viral respiratory infection in man. J Immunol 1970;105(3):584–91.

73. Russell CD, Unger SA, Walton M, et al. The human immune response to respiratory syncytial virus infection. Clin Microbiol Rev 2017;30(2):481–502.

74. Levandowski RA, Ou DW, Jackson GG. Acute-phase decrease of T lymphocyte subsets in rhinovirus infection. J Infect Dis 1986;153(4):743–8.

75. Connors TJ, Baird SJ, Yopes MC, et al. Developmental regulation of effector and resident memory T cell generation during pediatric viral respiratory tract infection. J Immunol 2018;201(2):432–9.

76. Heinonen S, Jartti T, Garcia C, et al. Rhinovirus detection in symptomatic and asymptomatic children value of host transcriptome analysis. Am J Respir Crit Care Med 2016;193(7):772–82.

77. Jartti T, Paul-Anttila M, Lehtinen P, et al. Systemic T-helper and T-regulatory cell type cytokine responses in rhinovirus vs. respiratory syncytial virus induced early wheezing: an observational study. Respir Res 2009;10:85.

78. Joshi P, Shaw A, Kakakios A, et al. Interferon-gamma levels in nasopharyngeal secretions of infants with respiratory syncytial virus and other respiratory viral infections. Clin Exp Immunol 2003;131(1):143–7.

79. Pinto RA, Arredondo SM, Bono MR, et al. T helper 1/T helper 2 cytokine imbalance in respiratory syncytial virus infection is associated with increased endogenous plasma cortisol. Pediatrics 2006;117(5):e878–86.

80. Bont L, Heijnen CJ, Kavelaars A, et al. Monocyte IL-10 production during respiratory syncytial virus bronchiolitis is associated with recurrent wheezing in a one-year follow-up study. Am J Respir Crit Care Med 2000;161(5):1518–23.

81. Mukherjee S, Lindell DM, Berlin AA, et al. IL-17-induced pulmonary pathogenesis during respiratory viral infection and exacerbation of allergic disease. Am J Pathol 2011;179(1):248–58.

82. Mangodt TC, Van Herck MA, Nullens S, et al. The role of Th17 and Treg responses in the pathogenesis of RSV infection. Pediatr Res 2015;78(5):483–91.

83. Wiehler S, Proud D. Interleukin-17A modulates human airway epithelial responses to human rhinovirus infection. Am J Physiol Lung Cell Mol Physiol 2007;293(2):L505–15.

84. Faber TE, Groen H, Welfing M, et al. Specific increase in local IL-17 production during recovery from primary RSV bronchiolitis. J Med Virol 2012;84(7):1084–8.

85. Durant LR, Makris S, Voorburg CM, et al. Regulatory T cells prevent Th2 immune responses and pulmonary eosinophilia during respiratory syncytial virus infection in mice. J Virol 2013;87(20):10946–54.

86. Ruckwardt TJ, Morabito KM, Graham BS. Determinants of early life immune responses to RSV infection. Curr Opin Virol 2016;16:151–7.

87. Martinez FD. Respiratory syncytial virus bronchiolitis and the pathogenesis of childhood asthma. Pediatr Infect Dis J 2003;22(2 Suppl):S76–82.

88. Crotty S. T follicular helper cell differentiation, function, and roles in disease. Immunity 2014;41(4):529–42.

89. Do LAH, Pellet J, van Doorn HR, et al. Host transcription profile in nasal epithelium and whole blood of hospitalized children under 2 years of age with respiratory syncytial virus infection. J Infect Dis 2017;217(1):134–46.

90. Kollmann TR, Kampmann B, Mazmanian SK, et al. Protecting the newborn and young infant from infectious diseases: lessons from immune ontogeny. Immunity 2017;46(3):350–63.

91. Restori KH, Srinivasa BT, Ward BJ, et al. Neonatal immunity, respiratory virus infections, and the development of asthma. Front Immunol 2018;9:1249.

92. Kollmann TR, Crabtree J, Rein-Weston A, et al. Neonatal innate TLR-mediated responses are distinct from those of adults. J Immunol 2009;183(11):7150–60.

93. Pedraza-Sánchez S, Hise AG, Ramachandra L, et al. Reduced frequency of a CD14+ CD16+ monocyte subset with high Toll-like receptor 4 expression in cord blood compared to adult blood contributes to lipopolysaccharide hyporesponsiveness in newborns. Clin Vaccine Immunol 2013;20(7):962–71.

94. Bucasas KL, Mian AI, Demmler-Harrison GJ, et al. Global gene expression profiling in infants with acute respiratory syncytial virus broncholitis demonstrates systemic activation of interferon signaling networks. Pediatr Infect Dis J 2013; 32(2):e68–76.

Bacteria in Asthma Pathogenesis

Michael Insel, MD[a], Monica Kraft, MD[b],*

KEYWORDS

- Asthma • Bacteria • Immunology • Microbiology

KEY POINTS

- Common atypical and nonatypical bacterial infections are associated with asthma symptoms and onset.
- Antibiotics mitigate asthma severity.
- The microbiome in infancy and adult life play an integral role in asthma pathogenesis and persistence.

INTRODUCTION

The airways are under continuous assault from aerosolized bacteria and oral flora. The bacteria present in the airways and gastrointestinal tract of neonates promote immune maturation and protect against asthma pathogenesis. Later bacterial infections and perturbations to the microbiome can contribute to asthma pathogenesis, persistence, and severity.

Many researchers initially believed that bacteria do not contribute to asthma because antibiotics did not seem to improve asthma symptoms.[1] Advances in bacterial identification and efforts to sample the airways directly led to the recognition that bacteria are critical to asthma pathogenesis. *Mycoplasma pneumoniae*, *Chlamydia pneumoniae*, *Chlamydia trachomatis*, *Staphylococcus aureus*, and *Haemophilus influenza* have all been identified as contributors to asthma. These findings led to a reexamination of the role of antibiotics in asthma with interesting results. More recently, advancements in profiling the respiratory microbiome continue to provide insights into the role commensal and pathogenic bacteria play in asthma pathogenesis.

Disclosure Statement: The authors have no commercial or financial conflicts of interest.
[a] Division of Pulmonary, Critical Care, Allergy, and Sleep Medicine, Department of Medicine, University of Arizona Health Sciences, University of Arizona College of Medicine – Tucson, 1501 North Campbell Avenue, PO Box 245017, Tucson, AZ 85724, USA; [b] Department of Medicine, College of Medicine Tucson, Asthma and Airway Disease Research Center, University of Arizona Health Sciences, University of Arizona College of Medicine – Tucson, 1501 North Campbell Avenue, PO Box 245017, Tucson, AZ 85724, USA
* Corresponding author.
E-mail address: kraftm@email.arizona.edu

MYCOPLASMA PNEUMONIAE

In 1984, Sabato and colleagues[2] found that 40% of children with acute *M pneumoniae* infection had wheezing. The nonasthmatic infected children had a persistent decrease in forced expiratory volume in 1 second. These findings raised the hypothesis that *M pneumoniae* could trigger the onset of asthma. Studies since have demonstrated that infection is associated with asthma exacerbations.[3,4] In fact, a higher IgM response in infection is associated with worse symptoms, indicating that the organism directly mediates asthma symptoms.[5] Chronic infection among asthmatics is also common[6,7] and is associated with worse daily symptoms.[8] Asthma also impairs *M pneumoniae* clearance,[9] suggesting that there is feedback between the host and organism.

Pathogenesis

M pneumoniae is a filamentous obligate organism that lacks a cell wall.[10] It enters the airway in droplets and attaches to epithelial cells via protein adhesins.[11] The P1 adhesin protein interdigitates between cilia and propels the bacteria into the distal airways.[12] P1 adhesin with other lipoproteins are recognized by toll-like receptors (TLR), which activate nuclear factor-κB and lead to tumor necrosis factor (TNF)-alpha,[13] IL-1beta,[14] and IL-8 release.[15] Community-acquired respiratory distress syndrome (CARDS) toxin, an ADP-ribosylating toxin, then traverses the host cell and promotes an IL-1 and TNF-alpha response,[16] causing vacuolization, cytoplasmic swelling, ciliostasis, and cell death.[16]

Wheezing in acute infection is associated with elevations in TLR2, TNF-alpha, IgE,[17] IL-10,[18] IL-5,[19] IL-4,[20] endothelin 1,[21] vascular endothelial growth factor,[22] and P1-specific IgE,[23] as well as reductions in IFN-gamma[17] and IL-18.[24]

In chronic and recurrent infection, both P1 adhesin and CARDS toxin can promote a type 2 inflammatory response. P1 adhesin activates mast cell release of IL-4 leading to B-cell IgE class switching.[25] CARDS toxin increases levels of type 2 cytokines[26] and can elicit its own IgE antibody response[28] (**Fig. 1**).

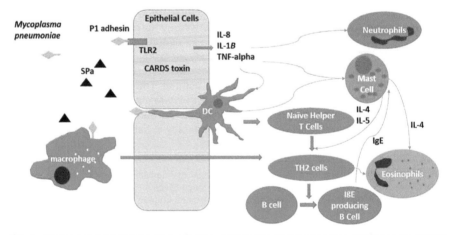

Fig. 1. *M pneumoniae* innate and adaptive immunity. *M pneumoniae* mediates an innate immune response via P1 adhesion TLR2 interaction on airway epithelial cells and dendritic cells (DC) and CARDS toxin inflammasome activation. There are subsequent increases in mast cell activation and neutrophil chemotaxis. Mast cell cytokine release in concert with dendritic cell activation leads to t cell class switching and promotion of type 2 inflammation. Preexisting atopy potentiates the TH2 response. Surfactant protein A (SP-A) can mitigate the inflammatory cascade.

Host Factors

Host factors mediate the asthmatic response to *M pneumoniae* infection. Asthmatic patients have a type 2 response after infection marked by increases in eosinophilic degranulation,[27] vascular endothelial growth factor, IL-5,[29] IL-4/13,[30] and dendritic cell Th2 priming.[31] Infection can also lead to increases in IL-17,[32] and decreases in IL-10 and IL-18,[33] indicative of non–type 2 inflammation.

Preexisting atopy increases the risk of asthma after infection.[34] Infected ovalbumin-sensitized mice have increased IL-4 production compared with nonsensitized mice.[35] Exposure to CARDS toxin alone leads to increased IL-4 and IL-13 in ovalbumin sensitized mice.[36] Sensitization also impairs *M pneumoniae* clearance via decreases in TLR2 and IL-6 expression.[32] Additionally, the short palate, lung, and nasal epithelium clone (SPLUNC1) protein a ubiquitous protein in the airways that assists with *M pneumoniae* clearance is downregulated in atopic disease.[33]

Surfactant protein A has a high affinity for *M pneumoniae*.[36] It inhibits eosinophil release of eosinophil peroxidase[37] and can inhibit mast cell release of TNF-alpha.[38] Surfactant protein A knockout mice have greater mucin production and neutrophil recruitment after infection. Defects in *M pneumoniae* binding are conferred by the SPA hSP-A2 223Q allele, a common human variant.[39,40]

Genetic variations in TNF-alpha, IL-1-beta,[41] and TLR2[42]—known mediators of the innate immune response in *M pneumoniae* infection—are associated with atopy and asthma severity. An impaired TLR2–IFN-gamma response can lead to an exuberant mucin response.[42]

Bacterial load and recurrent infection lead to an exuberant immune response that can vary depending on the amount of exposure. A high *M pneumoniae* bacterial load is associated with decreased IL-4 and eotaxin 2, whereas a chronic low-level load is associated with increased expression.[43] Repeated *M pneumoniae* infections are associated with elevations in IL-17, keratinocyte-derived cytokine, TNF-alpha, and IL-6 compared with a single exposure.[44] These findings suggests that persistent low-level exposures are responsible for a type 2 asthma phenotype, whereas recurrent infections may promote a Th17 phenotype.

CHLAMYDIA PNEUMONIAE
Pathogenesis

C pneumoniae enters the airway via droplets as nonreproductive elementary bodies and binds to epithelial cells. Once bound, it is phagocytosed into a protected double membrane inclusion body and evolves into a metabolically active reticulate body.[45] Virulence is partially mediated by the release of heat shock protein 60, which binds TLR2 and TLR4 leading to keratinocyte chemotaxis and IL-12 release, with subsequent neutrophil accumulation.[46] After multiple replications, the reticulate bodies convert back to an elementary body and induce cell death with bacterial exocytosis.[45]

Epidemiologic Studies

Forty-seven percent of patients with acute *C pneumoniae* infection have wheezing.[47] Asthmatics have a modestly increased *C pneumoniae* prevalence compared with controls measured by serology or polymerase chain reaction.[47] Although active infection is uncommon, in 1 study 79% of adults with severe asthma had heat shock protein 60 antibodies[48] and in another 50% had *C pneumoniae*–specific IgE present.[49] These data reveal that active colonization is incompletely detected by serology or polymerase chain reaction, or that asthmatics maintain a chronic immune reaction even after resolution of infection.

Asthma Phenotypes and C pneumoniae

C pneumoniae is associated with neutrophilic, chronic obstructive, and steroid-resistant asthma phenotypes. Asthmatic children with infection have a neutrophilic phenotype with increased IL-8 expression and BAL neutrophilia[50] mediated by increased IL-1-beta release via activation of the GTPase Rac 1[51] and increases in IL-12, IL-17, and IFN-gamma.[52]

Age of infection, previous allergen sensitization, and reinfection drive the phenotype. Mice infected as infants have increased IL-13 expression, mucus-secreting cells, and airway hyperresponsiveness, consistent with a type 2 phenotype. Meanwhile mice infected at birth have decreases in type 2 cytokines and dendritic cell numbers.[53] Age at infection also leads to differences in bone marrow dendritic cell programming.[54]

Allergen sensitization also affects phenotype. Among ova-sensitized mice, neonatal infection with *C pneumoniae* induces type 2 cytokines with associated chlamydia-specific IgE.[55] In contrast, infection during adulthood in sensitized-mice is associated with increased IL-2 and IFN-gamma expression.[55]

Chronic infection is associated with an accelerated decrease in forced expiratory volume in 1 second[56] and forced expiratory volume in 1 second/forced vital capacity[57] in both asthma and chronic obstructive pulmonary disease[58] and subepithelial basement membrane thickening on pathology.[59] Remodeling occurs via increases in monocyte expression of metalloproteinase-9 and tissue inhibitor metalloproteinase-1. Interestingly, infection also increases glucocorticoid receptor β expression, leading to increased steroid resistance.[60]

Not everyone with *C pneumoniae* develops chronic infection and asthma symptoms. CD14 and IL-6 polymorphisms are associated with macrophage bacterial clearance.[61] It remains unknown whether these differences mediate the asthmatic response to infection. TLR2 activation also promotes bacterial clearance via TNF-alpha and IL-1-beta release.[62] Plasmacytoid dendritic cells further help to maintain immunologic homeostasis after infection via CD4 cell chemotaxis and IL-10 release.[63] Plasmacytoid dendritic cell depletion is associated with chronic inflammation in mice. Further work is needed to elucidate the role of *C pneumoniae* in asthma pathogenesis.

CHLAMYDIA TRACHOMATIS

C trachomatis is associated with a type 2 asthma phenotype in children.[50,64] Allergen sensitization and reinfection promote a type 2 immune response. Bone marrow derived cells from mice infected with *Chlamydia muridarum*—a murine pathogen like *C trachomatis*—after ova sensitization have increased expression of innate and type 2 cytokines.[65] Acute *C muridarum* infection leads to increased IL-17 expression whereas reinfection promotes IL-17E (IL-25) expression[66]—a driver of type 2 inflammation.[67]

HAEMOPHILUS INFLUENZA

H influenza colonization is associated with neutrophilic asthma[68] and IL-17 expression.[69] Lipopolysaccharides in general have been shown to cause a shift toward neutrophilic inflammation in ova-sensitized mice.[70] Those with preexisting atopy show impaired *H influenza* clearance.[71] Furthermore, individuals with chronic allergic bronchitis have increased histamine release after *H influenza* exposure demonstrating a positive feedback between infection and the type 2 response.[72]

STAPHYLOCOCCUS AUREUS

Elevated levels of staphylococcus enterotoxin IgE are seen in adolescent and nonatopic adult-onset type 2 asthma.[73,74] Asthma severity correlates with staphylococcus enterotoxin IgE levels.[75] Smoking augments the response.[76] S aureus also produces alpha-hemolysin, which induces eosinophil cell death, which is thought to contribute to airway hyperreactivity.[77] Impaired macrophage phagocytosis[78] and Muc5b deficiency help to mediate staphylococcus enterotoxin-associated asthma[79] (Fig. 2).

ANTIBIOTICS IN ASTHMA

Macrolides are associated with decreased airway hyperresponsiveness,[80] exacerbation frequency and severity,[81] and steroid requirements,[82] as well as an improved quality of life.[83] Most of our current evidence suggests that macrolides work via immunomodulation rather than bacterial load reduction. They have been associated with reductions in IgE and IL-4 levels after C pneumoniae infection without affecting C pneumoniae copy number,[84] decreases in IL-13 and MUC5AC production,[85] and a decrease in IL-17 levels.[86] Even among asthmatics with acute rhinoviral infection, clarithromycin led to a decrease in IL-1-beta and IL-6 levels.[87] There is more recent evidence that macrolides alter the airway microbiome profile.[88]

THE MICROBIOME AND ASTHMA

In 1989, David Strachan observed that children in larger family units had lower incidence of hay fever,[89] prompting his proposal of the hygiene hypothesis—that early

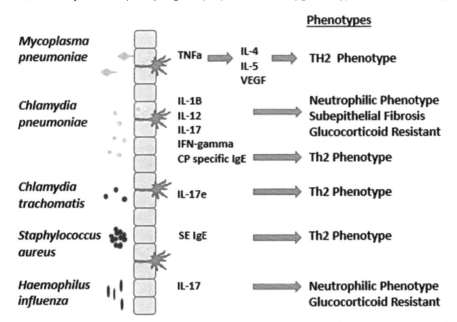

Fig. 2. The role of different bacterial infections in distinct asthma phenotypes. The role of different bacterial infections in distinct asthma phenotypes. *M pneumoniae, C pneumoniae* (CP), *C trachomatis,* and *S aureus*—via staphylococcus enterotoxin (SE)—have all been associated with the type 2 asthma phenotype (TH2). *C pneumoniae* and *H influenza* are primarily associated with a neutrophilic, glucocorticoid-resistant phenotype.

life exposures decrease risk of atopy. Follow-up studies demonstrated that increased endotoxin exposure was inversely associated with asthma and cytokine levels in children.[90] These findings inspired researchers to examine how the airway microbiome contributes to asthma pathogenesis.

The analysis of the microbiome in asthma pathogenesis has unique challenges. First, there is not a consensus on which microbiome matters most. Different segments of the respiratory system have unique microbial environments, and each segment has the risk of contamination from other segments.[91] Although the bronchi and bronchioles would seem to matter most in asthma pathogenesis, many immune cells in the airway originate in the bone marrow where they are preprogrammed. In addition, the gastrointestinal tract microbiome may have equal importance owing to immune cell priming and microaspiration.[92]

Another challenge is deciding what microbial community differences are pathologically meaningful when there is significant variation among phenotypically similar individuals. In addition, most studies to date have not answered whether unique airway microbial environments reflect or mediate immune function.

Neonatal Dysbiosis and Asthma

Neonatal colonization with *Streptococcus pneumoniae*, *Moraxella catarrhalis*, and *H influenza* predicts asthma risk.[93] *M catarrhalis* and *H influenza* are associated with a Th1/Th2/Th17 immune response and *S aureus* is associated with a TH17 response in neonates.[93] Colonization develops from maternal transmission, inherited immune dysfunction,[94] and possibly from the direct effect of antibiotics used by the mother. Questions remain over whether neonatal dysbiosis mediates asthma pathogenesis or if it reflects impaired immune function alone.[95]

Neonates with decreased gut microbial diversity have greater asthma risk. Decreased colonization of Lachnospira, Veillonella, Vaecalibacterium, and Rotha genera are associated with asthma.[96] Dysbiosis affects peripheral T-cell gene expression and subsequent atopy and asthma risk.[92] *Lactobacillus* supplementation may be able to reverse these effects.[97]

The Microbiome in Asthmatics

The phyla Firmicutes, Proteobacteria, Actinobacteria, Fusobacterium, and Bacteroides comprise more than 95% of the respiratory flora. The distribution across these phyla and the specific species composition differ between asthmatics and nonasthmatics and across asthma phenotypes. Nonasthmatics have more Firmicutes and Actinobacteria and asthmatics have a greater abundance of Proteobacteria.[98]

Asthmatic patients with sputum neutrophilia have less microbiologic diversity than those with eosinophilic or pauci-granulocytic phenotypes.[99] Sputum neutrophilia is associated with increased Moraxella and Haemophilus taxa[99] and Neisseria, Bacteroides, and Rothia species.[100] The TH17 asthma phenotype—noted for neutrophilia, severe symptoms, and corticosteroid insensitivity[101]—is associated with increased *Pasteurellaceae*, *Enterobacteriaceae*, and *Bacillaceae* families.[102]

Atopic asthmatics have greater phylogenetic diversity overall, but increases in type 2 cytokines are inversely correlated with total bacterial burden.[103] Streptomyces and Propionicimonas are specifically associated with bronchial biopsy eosinophilia[102]

Obese asthmatics with a predominately-adult onset phenotype demonstrate greater Bacteroidetes (specifically Prevotella) and Firmiticus species,[102] which may be explained by greater silent aspiration.[102]

Corticosteroid-resistant asthmatics have increases in gram negative bacteria with short length acyl lipid, a lipopolysaccharide (ie, *Haemophilus parainfleunza*). The short length lipopolysaccharide can activate transforming growth factor-β associated kinase and IL-8 release in a glucocorticoid receptor-independent pathway.[104] Interestingly, transforming growth factor-β associated kinase inhibition can restore corticosteroid sensitivity.[103] This potentially represents an exciting therapeutic path for patients with severe, steroid-resistant asthma if particular bacteria and their effects can be inhibited.

SUMMARY

Bacteria play a diverse and complex role in asthma pathogenesis. Acute and chronic exposures can precipitate asthma exacerbations and contribute to asthma persistence. Multiple host factors are essential to mediating an asthmatic immune response. The study of the microbiome in asthma provides new potential therapeutic targets.

REFERENCES

1. Shapiro GG, Eggleston PA, Pierson WE, et al. Double-blind study of the effectiveness of a broad-spectrum antibiotic in status asthmaticus. Pediatrics 1974; 53(6):867–72.
2. Sabato AR, Martin AJ, Marmion BP, et al. Mycoplasma pneumoniae: acute illness, antibiotics, and subsequent pulmonary function. Arch Dis Child 1984; 59(11):1034–7.
3. Seggev JS, Lis I, Siman-Tov R, et al. Mycoplasma pneumoniae is a frequent cause of exacerbation of bronchial asthma in adults. Ann Allergy 1986;57(4): 263–5.
4. Biscardi S, Lorrot M, Marc E, et al. Mycoplasma pneumoniae and asthma in children. Clin Infect Dis 2004;38(10):1341–6.
5. Kassisse E, Garcia H, Prada L, et al. Prevalence of Mycoplasma pneumoniae infection in pediatric patients with acute asthma exacerbation. Arch Argent Pediatr 2018;116(3):179–85.
6. Martin RJ, Kraft M, Chu HW, et al. A link between chronic asthma and chronic infection. J Allergy Clin Immunol 2001;107(4):595–601.
7. Kraft M, Cassell GH, Henson JE, et al. Detection of Mycoplasma pneumoniae in the airways of adults with chronic asthma. Am J Respir Crit Care Med 1998; 158(3):998–1001.
8. Wood PR, Hill VL, Burks ML, et al. Mycoplasma pneumoniae in children with acute and refractory asthma. Ann Allergy Asthma Immunol 2013;110(5):334.e1.
9. Shin JE, Cheon BR, Shim JW, et al. Increased risk of refractory Mycoplasma pneumoniae pneumonia in children with atopic sensitization and asthma. Korean J Pediatr 2014;57(6):271–7.
10. Waites KB, Talkington DF. Mycoplasma pneumoniae and its role as a human pathogen. Clin Microbiol Rev 2004;17(4):728, table of contents.
11. Razin S. Mycoplasmas. In: Baron S, editor. Medical microbiology. Galveston (TX): The University of Texas Medical Branch at Galveston; 1996. p. NBK7637 [bookaccession].
12. Seto S, Kenri T, Tomiyama T, et al. Involvement of P1 adhesin in gliding motility of Mycoplasma pneumoniae as revealed by the inhibitory effects of antibody under optimized gliding conditions. J Bacteriol 2005;187(5):1875–7.
13. Shimizu T, Kida Y, Kuwano K. A dipalmitoylated lipoprotein from Mycoplasma pneumoniae activates NF-kappa B through TLR1, TLR2, and TLR6. J Immunol 2005;175(7):4641–6.

14. Shimizu T, Kida Y, Kuwano K. Cytoadherence-dependent induction of inflammatory responses by *Mycoplasma pneumoniae*. Immunology 2011;133(1):51–61.
15. Chmura K, Bai X, Nakamura M, et al. Induction of IL-8 by *Mycoplasma pneumoniae* membrane in BEAS-2B cells. Am J Physiol Lung Cell Mol Physiol 2008; 295(1):220.
16. Kannan TR, Baseman JB. ADP-ribosylating and vacuolating cytotoxin of *Mycoplasma pneumoniae* represents unique virulence determinant among bacterial pathogens. Proc Natl Acad Sci U S A 2006;103(17):6724–9.
17. Fan Q, Gu T, Li P, et al. Roles of T-cell immunoglobulin and mucin domain genes and toll-like receptors in wheezy children with *Mycoplasma pneumoniae* pneumonia. Heart Lung Circ 2016;25(12):1226–31.
18. Medjo B, Atanaskovic-Markovic M, Nikolic D, et al. Increased serum interleukin-10 but not interleukin-4 level in children with *Mycoplasma pneumoniae* pneumonia. J Trop Pediatr 2017;63(4):294–300.
19. Esposito S, Droghetti R, Bosis S, et al. Cytokine secretion in children with acute mycoplasma pneumoniae infection and wheeze. Pediatr Pulmonol 2002;34(2): 122–7.
20. Koh YY, Park Y, Lee HJ, et al. Levels of interleukin-2, interferon-gamma, and interleukin-4 in bronchoalveolar lavage fluid from patients with mycoplasma pneumonia: implication of tendency toward increased immunoglobulin E production. Pediatrics 2001;107(3):E39.
21. Chung HL, Kim SG, Shin IH. The relationship between serum endothelin (ET)-1 and wheezing status in the children with mycoplasma pneumoniae pneumonia. Pediatr Allergy Immunol 2006;17(4):285–90.
22. Choi IS, Byeon JH, Yoo Y, et al. Increased serum interleukin-5 and vascular endothelial growth factor in children with acute mycoplasma pneumonia and wheeze. Pediatr Pulmonol 2009;44(5):423–8.
23. Ye Q, Mao JH, Shu Q, et al. *Mycoplasma pneumoniae* induces allergy by producing P1-specific immunoglobulin E. Ann Allergy Asthma Immunol 2018; 121(1):90–7.
24. Chung HL, Shin JY, Ju M, et al. Decreased interleukin-18 response in asthmatic children with severe mycoplasma pneumoniae pneumonia. Cytokine 2011; 54(2):218–21.
25. Hoek KL, Duffy LB, Cassell GH, et al. A role for the *Mycoplasma pneumoniae* adhesin P1 in interleukin (IL)-4 synthesis and release from rodent mast cells. Microb Pathog 2005;39(4):149–58.
26. Maselli DJ, Medina JL, Brooks EG, et al. The immunopathologic effects of Mycoplasma pneumoniae and community-acquired respiratory distress syndrome toxin. A primate model. Am J Respir Cell Mol Biol 2018;58(2):253–60.
27. Kim JH, Cho TS, Moon JH, et al. Serial changes in serum eosinophil-associated mediators between atopic and non-atopic children after *Mycoplasma pneumoniae* pneumonia. Allergy Asthma Immunol Res 2014;6(5):428–33.
28. Medina JL, Brooks EG, Chaparro A, et al. *Mycoplasma pneumoniae* CARDS toxin elicits a functional IgE response in balb/c mice. PLoS One 2017;12(2): e0172447.
29. Jeong YC, Yeo MS, Kim JH, et al. *Mycoplasma pneumoniae* infection affects the serum levels of vascular endothelial growth factor and interleukin-5 in atopic children. Allergy Asthma Immunol Res 2012;4(2):92–7.
30. Ye Q, Xu XJ, Shao WX, et al. *Mycoplasma pneumoniae* infection in children is a risk factor for developing allergic diseases. ScientificWorldJournal 2014;2014: 986527.

31. Shao L, Cong Z, Li X, et al. Changes in levels of IL-9, IL-17, IFN-gamma, dendritic cell numbers and TLR expression in peripheral blood in asthmatic children with mycoplasma pneumoniae infection. Int J Clin Exp Pathol 2015;8(5): 5263–72.

32. Wu Q, Martin RJ, Lafasto S, et al. Toll-like receptor 2 down-regulation in established mouse allergic lungs contributes to decreased mycoplasma clearance. Am J Respir Crit Care Med 2008;177(7):720–9.

33. Gally F, Di YP, Smith SK, et al. SPLUNC1 promotes lung innate defense against *Mycoplasma pneumoniae* infection in mice. Am J Pathol 2011;178(5):2159–67.

34. Yeh JJ, Wang YC, Hsu WH, et al. Incident asthma and *Mycoplasma pneumoniae*: a nationwide cohort study. J Allergy Clin Immunol 2016;137(4):1023.e6.

35. Chu HW, Honour JM, Rawlinson CA, et al. Effects of respiratory *Mycoplasma pneumoniae* infection on allergen-induced bronchial hyperresponsiveness and lung inflammation in mice. Infect Immun 2003;71(3):1520–6.

36. Medina JL, Coalson JJ, Brooks EG, et al. *Mycoplasma pneumoniae* CARDS toxin exacerbates ovalbumin-induced asthma-like inflammation in BALB/c mice. PLoS One 2014;9(7):e102613.

37. Ledford JG, Mukherjee S, Kislan MM, et al. Surfactant protein-A suppresses eosinophil-mediated killing of *Mycoplasma pneumoniae* in allergic lungs. PLoS One 2012;7(2):e32436.

38. Hsia BJ, Ledford JG, Potts-Kant EN, et al. Mast cell TNF receptors regulate responses to *Mycoplasma pneumoniae* in surfactant protein A (SP-A)-/- mice. J Allergy Clin Immunol 2012;130(1):14.e2.

39. Wang Y, Voelker DR, Lugogo NL, et al. Surfactant protein A is defective in abrogating inflammation in asthma. Am J Physiol Lung Cell Mol Physiol 2011;301(4): 598.

40. Ledford JG, Voelker DR, Addison KJ, et al. Genetic variation in SP-A2 leads to differential binding to *Mycoplasma pneumoniae* membranes and regulation of host responses. J Immunol 2015;194(12):6123–32.

41. Padron-Morales J, Sanz C, Davila I, et al. Polymorphisms of the IL12B, IL1B, and TNFA genes and susceptibility to asthma. J Investig Allergol Clin Immunol 2013; 23(7):487–94.

42. Wu Q, Martin RJ, Rino JG, et al. A deficient TLR2 signaling promotes airway mucin production in *Mycoplasma pneumoniae*-infected allergic mice. Am J Physiol Lung Cell Mol Physiol 2007;292(5):1064.

43. Wu Q, Martin RJ, LaFasto S, et al. A low dose of *Mycoplasma pneumoniae* infection enhances an established allergic inflammation in mice: the role of the prostaglandin E2 pathway. Clin Exp Allergy 2009;39(11):1754–63.

44. Kurai D, Nakagaki K, Wada H, et al. *Mycoplasma pneumoniae* extract induces an IL-17-associated inflammatory reaction in murine lung: implication for mycoplasmal pneumonia. Inflammation 2013;36(2):285–93.

45. Elwell C, Mirrashidi K, Engel J. Chlamydia cell biology and pathogenesis. Nat Rev Microbiol 2016;14(6):385–400.

46. Da Costa CU, Wantia N, Kirschning CJ, et al. Heat shock protein 60 from *Chlamydia pneumoniae* elicits an unusual set of inflammatory responses via toll-like receptor 2 and 4 in vivo. Eur J Immunol 2004;34(10):2874–84.

47. Hahn DL, Dodge RW, Golubjatnikov R. Association of *Chlamydia pneumoniae* (strain TWAR) infection with wheezing, asthmatic bronchitis, and adult-onset asthma. JAMA 1991;266(2):225–30.

48. Hahn DL, Peeling RW. Airflow limitation, asthma, and *Chlamydia pneumoniae*-specific heat shock protein 60. Ann Allergy Asthma Immunol 2008;101(6): 614–8.

49. Hahn DL, Schure A, Patel K, et al. *Chlamydia pneumoniae*-specific IgE is prevalent in asthma and is associated with disease severity. PLoS One 2012;7(4): e35945.

50. Patel KK, Vicencio AG, Du Z, et al. Infectious *Chlamydia pneumoniae* is associated with elevated interleukin-8 and airway neutrophilia in children with refractory asthma. Pediatr Infect Dis J 2010;29(12):1093–8.

51. Eitel J, Meixenberger K, van Laak C, et al. Rac1 regulates the NLRP3 inflammasome which mediates IL-1beta production in *Chlamydophila pneumoniae* infected human mononuclear cells. PLoS One 2012;7(1):e30379.

52. Horvat JC, Starkey MR, Kim RY, et al. Chlamydial respiratory infection during allergen sensitization drives neutrophilic allergic airways disease. J Immunol 2010;184(8):4159–69.

53. Horvat JC, Starkey MR, Kim RY, et al. Early-life chlamydial lung infection enhances allergic airways disease through age-dependent differences in immunopathology. J Allergy Clin Immunol 2010;125(3):625.e6.

54. Starkey MR, Kim RY, Beckett EL, et al. *Chlamydia muridarum* lung infection in infants alters hematopoietic cells to promote allergic airway disease in mice. PLoS One 2012;7(8):e42588.

55. Patel KK, Webley WC. Evidence of infectious asthma phenotype: chlamydia-induced allergy and pathogen-specific IgE in a neonatal mouse model. PLoS One 2013;8(12):e83453.

56. Pasternack R, Huhtala H, Karjalainen J. *Chlamydophila (chlamydia) pneumoniae* serology and asthma in adults: a longitudinal analysis. J Allergy Clin Immunol 2005;116(5):1123–8.

57. ten Brinke A, van Dissel JT, Sterk PJ, et al. Persistent airflow limitation in adult-onset nonatopic asthma is associated with serologic evidence of *Chlamydia pneumoniae* infection. J Allergy Clin Immunol 2001;107(3):449–54.

58. Droemann D, Rupp J, Goldmann T, et al. Disparate innate immune responses to persistent and acute *Chlamydia pneumoniae* infection in chronic obstructive pulmonary disease. Am J Respir Crit Care Med 2007;175(8):791–7.

59. Chen CZ, Yang BC, Lin TM, et al. Chronic and repeated *Chlamydophila pneumoniae* lung infection can result in increasing IL-4 gene expression and thickness of airway subepithelial basement membrane in mice. J Formos Med Assoc 2009;108(1):45–52.

60. Park CS, Lee YS, Kwon HS, et al. *Chlamydophila pneumoniae* inhibits corticosteroid-induced suppression of metalloproteinase-9 and tissue inhibitor metalloproteinase-1 secretion by human peripheral blood mononuclear cells. J Med Microbiol 2012;61(Pt 5):705–11.

61. Poikonen K, Lajunen T, Silvennoinen-Kassinen S, et al. Effects of CD14, TLR2, TLR4, LPB, and IL-6 gene polymorphisms on *Chlamydia pneumoniae* growth in human macrophages in vitro. Scand J Immunol 2009;70(1):34–9.

62. Netea MG, Kullberg BJ, Galama JM, et al. Non-LPS components of *Chlamydia pneumoniae* stimulate cytokine production through toll-like receptor 2-dependent pathways. Eur J Immunol 2002;32(4):1188–95.

63. Joyee AG, Yang X. Plasmacytoid dendritic cells mediate the regulation of inflammatory type T cell response for optimal immunity against respiratory *Chlamydia pneumoniae* infection. PLoS One 2013;8(12):e83463.

64. Webley WC, Tilahun Y, Lay K, et al. Occurrence of *Chlamydia trachomatis* and chlamydia pneumoniae in paediatric respiratory infections. Eur Respir J 2009; 33(2):360–7.
65. Kaiko GE, Phipps S, Hickey DK, et al. *Chlamydia muridarum* infection subverts dendritic cell function to promote Th2 immunity and airways hyperreactivity. J Immunol 2008;180(4):2225–32.
66. Mosolygo T, Spengler G, Endresz V, et al. IL-17E production is elevated in the lungs of balb/c mice in the later stages of *Chlamydia muridarum* infection and re-infection. In Vivo 2013;27(6):787–92.
67. Zhang X, Angkasekwinai P, Dong C, et al. Structure and function of interleukin-17 family cytokines. Protein Cell 2011;2(1):26–40.
68. Wood LG, Simpson JL, Hansbro PM, et al. Potentially pathogenic bacteria cultured from the sputum of stable asthmatics are associated with increased 8-isoprostane and airway neutrophilia. Free Radic Res 2010;44(2):146–54.
69. Essilfie AT, Simpson JL, Horvat JC, et al. *Haemophilus influenzae* infection drives IL-17-mediated neutrophilic allergic airways disease. PLoS Pathog 2011;7(10):e1002244.
70. Zhao S, Jiang Y, Yang X, et al. Lipopolysaccharides promote a shift from Th2-derived airway eosinophilic inflammation to Th17-derived neutrophilic inflammation in an ovalbumin-sensitized murine asthma model. J Asthma 2017;54(5): 447–55.
71. Essilfie AT, Simpson JL, Dunkley ML, et al. Combined haemophilus influenzae respiratory infection and allergic airways disease drives chronic infection and features of neutrophilic asthma. Thorax 2012;67(7):588–99.
72. Clementsen P, Milman N, Kilian M, et al. Endotoxin from haemophilus influenzae enhances IgE-mediated and non-immunological histamine release. Allergy 1990;45(1):10–7.
73. Song WJ, Sintobin I, Sohn KH, et al. Staphylococcal enterotoxin IgE sensitization in late-onset severe eosinophilic asthma in the elderly. Clin Exp Allergy 2016; 46(3):411–21.
74. Bachert C, van Steen K, Zhang N, et al. Specific IgE against Staphylococcus aureus enterotoxins: an independent risk factor for asthma. J Allergy Clin Immunol 2012;130(2):81.e8.
75. Kowalski ML, Cieslak M, Perez-Novo CA, et al. Clinical and immunological determinants of severe/refractory asthma (SRA): association with staphylococcal superantigen-specific IgE antibodies. Allergy 2011;66(1):32–8.
76. Nagasaki T, Matsumoto H, Oguma T, et al. Sensitization to staphylococcus aureus enterotoxins in smokers with asthma. Ann Allergy Asthma Immunol 2017;119(5):414.e2.
77. Prince LR, Graham KJ, Connolly J, et al. Staphylococcus aureus induces eosinophil cell death mediated by alpha-hemolysin. PLoS One 2012;7(2):e31506.
78. Liang Z, Zhang Q, Thomas CM, et al. Impaired macrophage phagocytosis of bacteria in severe asthma. Respir Res 2014;15:72.
79. Roy MG, Livraghi-Butrico A, Fletcher AA, et al. Muc5b is required for airway defence. Nature 2014;505(7483):412–6.
80. Kostadima E, Tsiodras S, Alexopoulos EI, et al. Clarithromycin reduces the severity of bronchial hyperresponsiveness in patients with asthma. Eur Respir J 2004;23(5):714–7.
81. Brusselle GG, Vanderstichele C, Jordens P, et al. Azithromycin for prevention of exacerbations in severe asthma (AZISAST): a multicentre randomised double-blind placebo-controlled trial. Thorax 2013;68(4):322–9.

82. Nelson HS, Hamilos DL, Corsello PR, et al. A double-blind study of troleandomycin and methylprednisolone in asthmatic subjects who require daily corticosteroids. Am Rev Respir Dis 1993;147(2):398–404.

83. Gibson PG, Yang IA, Upham JW, et al. Effect of azithromycin on asthma exacerbations and quality of life in adults with persistent uncontrolled asthma (AMAZES): a randomised, double-blind, placebo-controlled trial. Lancet 2017; 390(10095):659–68.

84. Dzhindzhikhashvili MS, Joks R, Smith-Norowitz T, et al. Doxycycline suppresses chlamydia pneumoniae-mediated increases in ongoing immunoglobulin E and interleukin-4 responses by peripheral blood mononuclear cells of patients with allergic asthma. J Antimicrob Chemother 2013;68(10):2363–8.

85. Mertens TC, Hiemstra PS, Taube C. Azithromycin differentially affects the IL-13-induced expression profile in human bronchial epithelial cells. Pulm Pharmacol Ther 2016;39:14–20.

86. An TJ, Rhee CK, Kim JH, et al. Effects of macrolide and corticosteroid in neutrophilic asthma mouse model. Tuberc Respir Dis (Seoul) 2018;81(1):80–7.

87. Yamaya M, Nomura K, Arakawa K, et al. Clarithromycin decreases rhinovirus replication and cytokine production in nasal epithelial cells from subjects with bronchial asthma: effects on IL-6, IL-8 and IL-33. Arch Pharm Res 2017.

88. Slater M, Rivett DW, Williams L, et al. The impact of azithromycin therapy on the airway microbiota in asthma. Thorax 2014;69(7):673–4.

89. Strachan DP. Hay fever, hygiene, and household size. BMJ 1989;299(6710): 1259–60.

90. Ege MJ, Mayer M, Normand AC, et al. Exposure to environmental microorganisms and childhood asthma. N Engl J Med 2011;364(8):701–9.

91. Durack J, Huang YJ, Nariya S, et al. Bacterial biogeography of adult airways in atopic asthma. Microbiome 2018;6(1):3.

92. Fujimura KE, Sitarik AR, Havstad S, et al. Neonatal gut microbiota associates with childhood multisensitized atopy and T cell differentiation. Nat Med 2016; 22(10):1187–91.

93. Bisgaard H, Hermansen MN, Buchvald F, et al. Childhood asthma after bacterial colonization of the airway in neonates. N Engl J Med 2007;357(15):1487–95.

94. Folsgaard NV, Schjorring S, Chawes BL, et al. Pathogenic bacteria colonizing the airways in asymptomatic neonates stimulates topical inflammatory mediator release. Am J Respir Crit Care Med 2013;187(6):589–95.

95. Stokholm J, Sevelsted A, Bonnelykke K, et al. Maternal propensity for infections and risk of childhood asthma: a registry-based cohort study. Lancet Respir Med 2014;2(8):631–7.

96. Arrieta MC, Stiemsma LT, Dimitriu PA, et al. Early infancy microbial and metabolic alterations affect risk of childhood asthma. Sci Transl Med 2015;7(307): 307ra152.

97. Yu J, Jang SO, Kim BJ, et al. The effects of lactobacillus rhamnosus on the prevention of asthma in a murine model. Allergy Asthma Immunol Res 2010;2(3): 199–205.

98. Marri PR, Stern DA, Wright AL, et al. Asthma-associated differences in microbial composition of induced sputum. J Allergy Clin Immunol 2013;131(2):3.

99. Taylor SL, Leong LEX, Choo JM, et al. Inflammatory phenotypes in patients with severe asthma are associated with distinct airway microbiology. J Allergy Clin Immunol 2018;141(1):103.e15.

100. Sverrild A, Kiilerich P, Brejnrod A, et al. Eosinophilic airway inflammation in asthmatic patients is associated with an altered airway microbiome. J Allergy Clin Immunol 2017;140(2):417.e11.

101. Furukawa T, Sakagami T, Koya T, et al. Characteristics of eosinophilic and non-eosinophilic asthma during treatment with inhaled corticosteroids. J Asthma 2015;52(4):417–22.

102. Huang YJ, Nariya S, Harris JM, et al. The airway microbiome in patients with severe asthma: associations with disease features and severity. J Allergy Clin Immunol 2015;136(4):874–84.

103. Durack J, Lynch SV, Nariya S, et al. Features of the bronchial bacterial microbiome associated with atopy, asthma, and responsiveness to inhaled corticosteroid treatment. J Allergy Clin Immunol 2017;140(1):63–75.

104. Goleva E, Jackson LP, Harris JK, et al. The effects of airway microbiome on corticosteroid responsiveness in asthma. Am J Respir Crit Care Med 2013;188(10): 1193–201.

Beyond Respiratory Syncytial Virus and Rhinovirus in the Pathogenesis and Exacerbation of Asthma

The Role of Metapneumovirus, Bocavirus and Influenza Virus

Andrea M. Coverstone, MD[a], Leyao Wang, PhD, MPH[b],
Kaharu Sumino, MD, MPH[c],*

KEYWORDS

- Human metapneumovirus • Bocavirus • Influenza virus • Wheezing • Asthma

KEY POINTS

- Respiratory viruses other than rhinovirus or respiratory syncytial virus can be associated with acute wheezing illness.
- Contribution to recurrent/wheezing is not well studied.
- Children with human metapneumovirus lower respiratory tract infection may have increased risk of subsequent recurrent wheezing over the several years after initial infection.

With the dissemination of the use of sensitive molecular methods for viral detection, the opportunities to evaluate the role of respiratory viruses in acute and chronic respiratory illness has expanded in the past decade. Acute wheezing illnesses are common, especially in young children, and viral agents have been shown to be found in 60% to 100% of these episodes using these sensitive detection methods.[1–3] Multiple

Disclosure: The authors have no conflicts to report.
[a] Division of Allergy, Immunology and Pulmonary Medicine, Department of Pediatrics, Washington University School of Medicine, 1 Children's Place, Campus Box 8116, Saint Louis, MO 63110, USA; [b] Division of Pulmonary and Critical Care Medicine, Department of Medicine, Washington University School of Medicine, 425 S. Euclid Avenue, CB 8052, Saint Louis, MO 63110, USA; [c] Division of Pulmonary and Critical Care Medicine, Department of Medicine, Washington University School of Medicine, 660 Euclid Avenue, Campus Box 8052, Saint Louis, MO 63110, USA
* Corresponding author.
E-mail address: ksumino@wustl.edu

viruses are associated with acute wheezing illness, including rhinovirus (RV), respiratory syncytial virus (RSV), human metapneumovirus (hMPV), influenza virus, parainfluenza virus, adenovirus, human bocavirus (HBoV),[1] coronavirus, and enterovirus (**Table 1**). These viruses have also been shown to be associated with asthma exacerbations.[4,5] RV and RSV are the most frequently detected pathogens (see **Table 1**), with RSV more prevalent in younger children in winter months and RV more prevalent in older children.[2] There is a large body of evidence implicating the association of RV[6–8] and RSV[9,10] with the subsequent development of recurrent wheezing and/or asthma. Viruses other than RV or RSV can be detected in 50% of wheezing illnesses,[1,11,12] but there are limited data regarding the association of these other viruses and asthma. Conducting studies to evaluate the long-term consequences of these other viruses has been challenging for several reasons. First, the detection rate of these viruses is often lower compared with RV and RSV, so a much larger cohort is required to perform a study with adequate representation of patients infected with these other viruses. The prospective study that investigated the role of hMPV infection in the development of wheezing and asthma required screening of more than 400 children infected with hMPV over a 5-year period of recruitment.[13] Second, establishing appropriate animal models has been challenging and existing models may not adequately model human infection to evaluate long-term outcomes. Third, it is difficult to tease out the specific contribution of other viruses because the association of RV and RSV can confound the analysis given the high rate of coinfection with these viruses. For instance, in a community cohort of 147 children with high atopic risk, wheezy, febrile lower respiratory tract infection (LRTI) during the first year of life was associated with a higher risk of persistent wheezing (odds ratio [OR], 3.5) and asthma (OR, 4.9) at age 10 years if they were atopic by age 2 years.[3] Respiratory virus was detected in 62% of these patients with febrile LRTI with a large proportion (60%–70%) of the detected viruses being RV or RSV, so this observed association may be primarily caused by the effect of RV or RSV infection. However, there are data suggesting that viral infection in early life with any cause may be important in increasing the risk of asthma. In a high-risk birth cohort study in Demark, the number of respiratory episodes in the first year of life was associated with the development of asthma at age 7 years regardless of virus type.[14]

This article focuses on 3 viruses (hMPV, HBoV, and influenza virus) in which an association with wheezing illness has been most studied. It provides an aggregate of

Table 1
Frequency of viruses detected in acute wheezing illness in children

Virus	Frequency (%)
RV	28–76
RSV	16–29
Enterovirus	4–27
Bocavirus	5–18
Parainfluenza virus	8–9
HMPV	3–6
Adenovirus	3–7
Coronavirus	2–5
Influenza virus	2–4

Data from Refs.[1–3]

available data reviewing the current research investigating the role of these viruses in acute and chronic respiratory disease.

HUMAN BOCAVIRUS

hMPV is a paramyxovirus first discovered by van den Hoogen and colleagues[15] in 2001. Similar to RSV, hMPV is a single-stranded RNA virus belonging to the Pneumoviridae subfamily, and causes many of the same symptoms as RSV. Typical symptoms of hMPV infection include mild, self-limiting, acute upper respiratory tract infections to more severe LRTIs, with wheezing and pneumonia. It is a frequent cause of bronchiolitis in young children.[16] Cough, rhinorrhea, wheeze, and fever are commonly reported symptoms in children infected with hMPV.[17–22]

Virtually all children have evidence of exposure to hMPV by age 5 years.[15] hMPV is responsible for a significant portion (2%–12%) of respiratory tract infections[16,17,19,23–26] and is associated with a large burden of hospitalizations and outpatient visits in younger children.[18,20] It tends to peak during the late winter and spring seasons, typically between December and April,[16,19,22,24] often peaking in February and March. Compared with infection with other viruses, there have been conflicting data on whether hMPV infections result in greater hypoxemia or duration of hospitalization or intensive care unit (ICU) stays.[23,24] The severity of illness is worse in those with a history of extreme prematurity.[25]

Although hMPV causes wheezing and lower respiratory tract symptoms, the contribution of hMPV to asthma exacerbations varies among different populations. In those with asthma exacerbations, the detection rate of hMPV is approximately 5% worldwide,[4] whereas in those with hMPV LRTI a much higher proportion have a diagnosis of asthma. In a study of children with hMPV LRTIs in the United States, 14% to 33% carried a diagnosis of asthma or history of wheezing.[16,19] In a study of children with hMPV in Spain, 60.7% of those infected with hMPV alone carried a diagnosis of recurrent wheeze or asthma, which was higher than rates in RSV or adenovirus but similar to that of RV or HBoV. Children with RSV were more likely to have a diagnosis of bronchiolitis than children with hMPV.[24] hMPV can cause an illness consistent with bronchiolitis, but children may be diagnosed less often with this term, given that it often is synonymous with RSV infections in young children. Nonetheless, hMPV causes wheezing in young children; can often precipitate episodes of wheezing in those prone to do so, such as asthmatics; and is an important cause of viral-induced asthma exacerbations. In children with asthma, studies have shown synergistic effects of allergic characteristics of the host (ie, immunoglobulin E level, house dust sensitization) and the severity of asthma exacerbation by RV,[27,28] but the interaction of allergy of the host and hMPV infection has not been well studied.

In contrast with the large number of studies reporting the association of hMPV in early childhood with acute wheezing illnesses or asthma at the time of illness,[16,23] there are sparse data on the long-term consequences after the acute infection. One study from Garcia-Garcia and colleagues[26] retrospectively identified children 2 to 5 years of age who were hospitalized with hMPV or RSV bronchiolitis in their first 24 months of life and contacted them to assess their diagnosis of asthma at the time of the study. Of 101 children with hMPV-positive bronchiolitis (without coinfection) over the course of the prior 5 years (October 2000 to June 2005), they were able to obtain follow-up on 23 children with no prior history of wheezing. They then selected a random sample of children in that same time period with RSV bronchiolitis and obtained follow-up on 32 of those children. A diagnosis of recurrent wheezing and asthma was more frequent in children with a history of hMPV bronchiolitis or RSV bronchiolitis compared with control children who were hospitalized around the same time because of rotavirus. hMPV bronchiolitis was the strongest independent risk factor for asthma (OR, 15.9; confidence interval [CI], 3.6, 70.5), followed by RSV bronchiolitis (OR, 10.1; CI, 2.5, 40.1) and allergic rhinitis (OR, 4.9; CI, 1.2, 40.1) at age 3 to 5 years. Another study prospectively followed premature infants with viral LRTI and, although it did not track wheezing or asthma status, found that airway resistance measures were increased at 1 year of age, although this study included only 4 infants with hMPV.[29]

Stronger evidence for the long-term effect of hMPV LTRI was found in a recent prospective study that evaluated the effects of hMPV infection on wheezing and asthma outcomes. Children less than 5 years of age hospitalized or treated in the emergency room with hMPV LRTI and no prior history of wheezing were prospectively followed along with a control group, with outcome assessment every 3 to 6 months for up to 3 years, and a final follow-up as late as 6.5 years.[13] This prospective study design enabled the investigators to obtain the child's wheezing history and capture the outcome securely in a longitudinal fashion. Follow-up data were collected on 29 children with hPMV LRTI and 27 controls. Children with hMPV LRTI had a higher likelihood of wheezing episodes during the follow-up period (hazard ratio [HR], 2.8; CI, 1.4, 5.8) than controls. In addition, children with hMPV LRTI had earlier onset of recurrent wheezing, both with and without colds, than the control children (**Fig. 1**). The association with the development of asthma was not statistically significant (HR, 2.5; CI, 0.8, 8.1; $P = .12$), although the number of children diagnosed with asthma was larger in the hMPV group (9 of 29) than the control group (4 of 27). There is more to learn, but these studies suggest an increased risk of asthma development following hMPV infection early in life.

The mechanism of short-term and long-term pathologic effects of hMPV infection is not well studied compared with that of RSV. Infection with hMPV in mice was shown to lead to persistence of viral RNA, pulmonary inflammation, and airway hyperresponsiveness several months after the infection,[30] suggesting long-term pathologic changes can occur after hMPV infection.

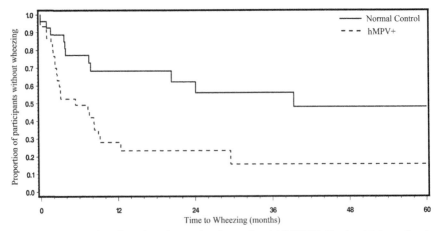

Fig. 1. Survival analysis for wheezing and asthma after hMPV LRTI. Kaplan-Meier estimates of freedom from any wheezing episodes, $P = .004$; hMPV LRTI subjects had wheezing earlier in follow-up compared with control subjects. (*From* Coverstone AM, Wilson B, Burgdorf D, et al. Recurrent wheezing in children following human metapneumovirus infection. J Allergy Clin Immunol 2018;142(1):299; with permission.)

Studies in both mice and humans have suggested several different molecular mechanisms of hMPV affect airway inflammation and function at the time of acute infection, often comparing these mechanisms with those of other viral causes. Alveolar macrophage activity may be augmented in hMPV infection, leading to detrimental effects on the airway, whereas alveolar macrophage depletion was seen in RSV and may provide protection against the harmful effects of the virus.[31] The chemokine profile of nasal secretions was also shown to differ in hMPV, with high concentrations of interleukin (IL)-8 (neutrophil chemotactic factor) and low concentrations of RANTES (regulated on activation, normal T-cell expressed and secreted) (eosinophil chemotactic factor) in individuals infected with hMPV compared with the increased RANTES concentrations seen in RSV.[17] In another study of children 1 to 14 years of age with hMPV infection, differences in measures of cell-mediated immunity distinguished hMPV from other respiratory viruses, such as RSV and influenza.[22] Thymic stromal lymphopoietin (TSLP) as well as IL-4 plasma levels were higher in children with wheezing and hMPV than in those without wheezing and hMPV or without wheezing and another respiratory virus. TSLP has been implicated as a mediator in the pathway of pediatric asthma, with higher plasma TSLP levels correlating with poor asthma control.[32] TSLP promotes basophil production and type 2 inflammation.[33] Infection of human airway epithelial cells with hMPV induced expression of TSLP, as well as leading to upregulation of IL-8 and IL-33, whereas TSLP blockade led to reduced lung inflammation,[34] indicating activation of the TSLP pathway initiating airway inflammation by hMPV acute infection. These studies may suggest the involvement of the TSLP pathway as a molecular mechanism for how hMPV leads to a recurrent wheezing and asthma phenotype, although further investigation is warranted.

HUMAN BOCAVIRUS

HBoV is a parvovirus that was discovered in 2005 from pooled nasopharyngeal samples by molecular screening.[35] Subsequent studies have shown that HBoV genotype 1 is commonly detected in respiratory samples from children with acute wheezing.[1,12] In children with acute wheezing for the first time, HBoV was detected in 18%.[12] However, it is also known that the coinfection rate of HBoV with other viruses is very high (15%–100%). In addition, detection in asymptomatic individuals is also frequent. HBoV was found to be present in 17% of healthy controls admitted to the hospital for elective surgery,[36] and in participants in a household study in which symptoms and nasal samples were prospectively collected for 12 months, 50% of HBoV detection occurred in those without symptoms.[37] Viral persistence is thought to be responsible for the high frequency of coinfection.[37,38] HBoV 1 is implicated to be an important respiratory pathogen by many,[39,40] but the precise pathologic contribution of HBoV in acute respiratory disease is still not accurately defined and HBoV may be both a passenger and a causative pathogen.[36,41] HBoV may interfere with RV-induced immune responses during acute wheezing. Lukkarinen and colleagues[42] compared the T-helper (Th) 1, Th2, proinflammatory cytokine response profile in young children with RV, HBoV, and RV-HBoV coinfection with acute wheezing illness. Unlike RV, HBoV infection was not associated with systemic proinflammatory or Th2-type responses and the RV-HBoV coinfection resulted in a non–Th2-type immune response.

Although bocavirus is frequently detected and seems to be associated with acute wheezing episodes, the data on long-term consequences after the acute infection are sparse. One retrospective study from Spain identified children who were previously hospitalized with HBoV (n = 10) or RSV bronchiolitis (n = 80) in their first 24 months of life and evaluated them to assess clinical outcomes, including a diagnosis of asthma and presence of atopy at age 5 to 7 years.[43] All children in the HBoV group developed recurrent wheezing. Fifty percent in the HBoV group and 23% in the RSV group had a diagnosis of asthma at age 5 to 7 years. The proportion of those with atopy was similar among those with HBoV and RSV. Another study in children hospitalized for acute viral wheezing showed that 13 children with HBoV-associated bronchiolitis had recurrent wheezing 2 years after the initial hospitalization less often than children with RV-associated bronchiolitis (HBoV 40% vs RV 60%).[42] The association of HBoV LRTI in early life and asthma is inconclusive and larger prospective studies are required to confirm these findings.

INFLUENZA VIRUS

Influenza viruses are responsible for an average of 3.1 million annual hospitalized days, and 31.4 million outpatient visits,[44] and is one of the frequently detected viruses during asthma exacerbations. It has long been identified as a precipitant of asthma exacerbations in all age groups.[2,4,45] In people with asthma exacerbations, the detection rate of influenza virus is approximately 10% worldwide,[4] but, during a flu season, the prevalence of influenza viruses can be as high as 20% in wheezing infants and 20% to 25% in adults with acute asthma exacerbations.[2,46,47] Although involvement of influenza virus is common in asthma exacerbation, influenza virus is an infrequent cause of acute wheezing illness in younger children.[1–3] The authors are not aware of any studies evaluating the role of influenza virus LRTI on the development of recurrent wheezing and/or asthma later in life.

The cytokine IL-33 is implicated as an important driver for influenza-induced asthma exacerbations in animal studies.[48,49] In the influenza-infected mouse models, IL-33 expression is upregulated, shifting the balance of Th1/Th2 immunity.[48,50] A recent study has shown that IL-33 is produced by ciliated bronchial cells and type II alveolar cells on viral-induced exacerbation in human and mice and dampened innate and adaptive Th1-like and cytotoxic responses, which subsequently results in increased viral loads and enhanced airway inflammation underlying the influenza-induced asthma exacerbation.[49] Meanwhile, heightened IL-33 production induces substantial IL-13 production in type 2 innate lymphoid cells (ILC-2), Th2 cytokine–producing cells that promote allergic inflammation in mouse models of asthma and atopic dermatitis.[51] In another study, influenza A infection induced acute airway hyperreactivity that was medicated by ILC-2, suggesting the importance of the IL-33–IL-13 axis in influenza-induced acute asthma exacerbations.[52]

Whether asthmatics are more frequently infected by influenza virus is still a matter of debate. It has been shown that patients with asthma have reduced type 1 interferon (IFN) responses on RV infection,[53,54] but a few studies did not confirm this observation.[55,56] Human bronchial epithelial cells from patients with asthma show increased IFN-lambda 1 levels and preserved IFN-beta levels when infected with influenza A virus, although viral levels were higher in asthmatics compared with nonasthmatics.[56] In a US study, children with asthma were found to be infected twice as often as nonasthmatics by H1N1 influenza when monitored by weekly nasal samples and symptoms scores during the 2009 to 2010 season.[57] Regardless, it has been accepted that asthma is a risk factor of severe disease with influenza once acquired, and patients with asthma have been listed as a priority population for vaccination.[58] The population studies in the 2009 H1N1 pandemic have provided interesting observations regarding this susceptibility. Having asthma was found to be a risk factor for hospitalization for H1N1[59,60] and was found in 10% to 20% of the hospitalized patients worldwide.[61] Nonetheless, an observation has also been made that having asthma may be protective once patients are hospitalized from influenza. Patients with asthma had decreased risk of ICU stay, mechanical ventilation, and death from H1N1, compared with other chronic conditions, such as cardiovascular diseases and obesity.[62–64] The observed protective effect may be in part explained by early hospital admission and/or a favorable response to steroids.[65] In mouse models, this protective effect of allergic asthma on influenza infection has been recapitulated and the increased eosinophil levels in asthmatic airways may be one of the mechanisms.[66] With putative antigen-presenting functions, eosinophils enhanced influenza-specific CD8+ T cells after infection, mediating the viral clearance of influenza virus in a mouse asthma model.[66] Rapid induction of type III IFNs, natural killer cells, and TGF-beta was also observed in asthmatic mice on influenza infection, indicating a potential mechanism for enhanced antiviral immunity against influenza in asthmatics.[66–68]

Influenza vaccine is recommended for patients with asthma in many countries, but there has not been clear evidence showing a protective benefit. The most recent Cochrane Review, in 2013, which included 18 trials across the world, concluded that inactivated influenza vaccine did not provide significant reduction in the number or duration of influenza-related asthma exacerbations.[69] Safety concern was raised in an earlier study that showed a decrease in peak flow following the administration of the inactivated influenza vaccine.[70] A subsequent study in the Netherlands[71] and a large study in the United States[72] enrolling more than 2000 patients with asthma confirmed that there is no increase in risk for adverse events including asthma exacerbation within 2 weeks following the injection. This Cochran Review also conducted a systematic review in 3 trials comparing intranasal vaccine with intramuscular infection in infants and older children and concluded that event rates for asthma exacerbation and wheezing were similar in both vaccine types.[69] A more recent study in the United Kingdom evaluated the safety of intranasal live attenuated influenza vaccine in atopic children with well-defined allergy to eggs. Sixty-seven percent of children had asthma in addition to their egg allergies. There was no systemic reaction following the injections and 8 mild self-limiting symptoms after 433 doses given in 282 children, which also ensured safety.[73]

SUMMARY

Respiratory viruses other than RV or RSV, especially hMPV, influenza virus, and HBoV, can be detected frequently in acute wheezing illness. The interaction of these other viruses with an allergic host, and their contribution in the development of asthma after acute infection, are not well understood, although there is evidence to suggest that children with hMPV LRTI have a higher likelihood of subsequent and recurrent wheezing over the several years after initial infection.

REFERENCES

1. Allander T, Jartti T, Gupta S, et al. Human bocavirus and acute wheezing in children. Clin Infect Dis 2007;44(7):904–10.
2. Heymann PW, Carper HT, Murphy DD, et al. Viral infections in relation to age, atopy, and season of admission among children hospitalized for wheezing. J Allergy Clin Immunol 2004;114(2):239–47.
3. Kusel MM, Kebadze T, Johnston SL, et al. Febrile respiratory illnesses in infancy and atopy are risk factors for persistent asthma and wheeze. Eur Respir J 2012; 39(4):876–82.

4. Zheng XY, Xu YJ, Guan WJ, et al. Regional, age and respiratory-secretion-specific prevalence of respiratory viruses associated with asthma exacerbation: a literature review. Arch Virol 2018;163(4):845–53.
5. Tan WC. Viruses in asthma exacerbations. Curr Opin Pulm Med 2005;11(1):21–6.
6. Rubner FJ, Jackson DJ, Evans MD, et al. Early life rhinovirus wheezing, allergic sensitization, and asthma risk at adolescence. J Allergy Clin Immunol 2017; 139(2):501–7.
7. Jackson DJ, Gangnon RE, Evans MD, et al. Wheezing rhinovirus illnesses in early life predict asthma development in high-risk children. Am J Respir Crit Care Med 2008;178(7):667–72.
8. Anderson HM, Lemanske RF Jr, Evans MD, et al. Assessment of wheezing frequency and viral etiology on childhood and adolescent asthma risk. J Allergy Clin Immunol 2017;139(2):692–4.
9. Bacharier LB, Cohen R, Schweiger T, et al. Determinants of asthma after severe respiratory syncytial virus bronchiolitis. J Allergy Clin Immunol 2012;130(1): 91–100 e103.
10. Sigurs N, Aljassim F, Kjellman B, et al. Asthma and allergy patterns over 18 years after severe RSV bronchiolitis in the first year of life. Thorax 2010;65(12):1045–52.
11. Kusel MM, de Klerk NH, Kebadze T, et al. Early-life respiratory viral infections, atopic sensitization, and risk of subsequent development of persistent asthma. J Allergy Clin Immunol 2007;119(5):1105–10.
12. Turunen R, Koistinen A, Vuorinen T, et al. The first wheezing episode: respiratory virus etiology, atopic characteristics, and illness severity. Pediatr Allergy Immunol 2014;25(8):796–803.
13. Coverstone AM, Wilson B, Burgdorf D, et al. Recurrent wheezing in children following human metapneumovirus infection. J Allergy Clin Immunol 2018; 142(1):297–301.e2.
14. Bonnelykke K, Vissing NH, Sevelsted A, et al. Association between respiratory infections in early life and later asthma is independent of virus type. J Allergy Clin Immunol 2015;136(1):81–6.e4.
15. van den Hoogen BG, de Jong JC, Groen J, et al. A newly discovered human pneumovirus isolated from young children with respiratory tract disease. Nat Med 2001;7(6):719–24.
16. Williams JV, Harris PA, Tollefson SJ, et al. Human metapneumovirus and lower respiratory tract disease in otherwise healthy infants and children. N Engl J Med 2004;350(5):443–50.
17. Jartti T, van den Hoogen B, Garofalo RP, et al. Metapneumovirus and acute wheezing in children. Lancet 2002;360(9343):1393–4.
18. Boivin G, De Serres G, Cote S, et al. Human metapneumovirus infections in hospitalized children. Emerg Infect Dis 2003;9(6):634–40.
19. Agapov E, Sumino KC, Gaudreault-Keener M, et al. Genetic variability of human metapneumovirus infection: evidence of a shift in viral genotype without a change in illness. J Infect Dis 2006;193(3):396–403.
20. Wei HY, Tsao KC, Huang CG, et al. Clinical features of different genotypes/genogroups of human metapneumovirus in hospitalized children. J Microbiol Immunol 2013;46(5):352–7.
21. Zhang L, Liu W, Liu D, et al. Epidemiological and clinical features of human metapneumovirus in hospitalised paediatric patients with acute respiratory illness: a cross-sectional study in Southern China, from 2013 to 2016. BMJ Open 2018; 8(2):e019308.

22. Gu W, Wang Y, Hao C, et al. Elevated serum levels of thymic stromal lymphopoietin in wheezing children infected with human metapneumovirus. Jpn J Infect Dis 2017;70(2):161–6.
23. Edwards KM, Zhu Y, Griffin MR, et al. Burden of human metapneumovirus infection in young children. N Engl J Med 2013;368(7):633–43.
24. Garcia-Garcia ML, Calvo C, Rey C, et al. Human metapnuemovirus infections in hospitalized children and comparison with other respiratory viruses. 2005-2014 prospective study. PLoS One 2017;12(3):e0173504.
25. Pancham K, Sami I, Perez GF, et al. Human metapneumovirus infection is associated with severe respiratory disease in preschool children with history of prematurity. Pediatr Neonatol 2016;57(1):27–34.
26. Garcia-Garcia ML, Calvo C, Casas I, et al. Human metapneumovirus bronchiolitis in infancy is an important risk factor for asthma at age 5. Pediatr Pulmonol 2007; 42(5):458–64.
27. Olenec JP, Kim WK, Lee WM, et al. Weekly monitoring of children with asthma for infections and illness during common cold seasons. J Allergy Clin Immunol 2010; 125(5):1001–6.e1.
28. Kantor DB, Stenquist N, McDonald MC, et al. Rhinovirus and serum IgE are associated with acute asthma exacerbation severity in children. J Allergy Clin Immunol 2016;138(5):1467–71.e9.
29. Broughton S, Sylvester KP, Fox G, et al. Lung function in prematurely born infants after viral lower respiratory tract infections. Pediatr Infect Dis J 2007;26(11): 1019–24.
30. Hamelin ME, Prince GA, Gomez AM, et al. Human metapneumovirus infection induces long-term pulmonary inflammation associated with airway obstruction and hyperresponsiveness in mice. J Infect Dis 2006;193(12):1634–42.
31. Kolli D, Gupta MR, Sbrana E, et al. Alveolar macrophages contribute to the pathogenesis of human metapneumovirus infection while protecting against respiratory syncytial virus infection. Am J Respir Cell Mol Biol 2014;51(4):502–15.
32. Chauhan A, Singh M, Agarwal A, et al. Correlation of TSLP, IL-33, and CD4 + CD25 + FOXP3 + T regulatory (Treg) in pediatric asthma. J Asthma 2015; 52(9):868–72.
33. Siracusa MC, Saenz SA, Hill DA, et al. TSLP promotes interleukin-3-independent basophil haematopoiesis and type 2 inflammation. Nature 2011;477(7363): 229–33.
34. Lay MK, Cespedes PF, Palavecino CE, et al. Human metapneumovirus infection activates the TSLP pathway that drives excessive pulmonary inflammation and viral replication in mice. Eur J Immunol 2015;45(6):1680–95.
35. Allander T, Tammi MT, Eriksson M, et al. Cloning of a human parvovirus by molecular screening of respiratory tract samples. Proc Natl Acad Sci U S A 2005; 102(36):12891–6.
36. Christensen A, Nordbo SA, Krokstad S, et al. Human bocavirus in children: monodetection, high viral load and viraemia are associated with respiratory tract infection. J Clin Virol 2010;49(3):158–62.
37. Byington CL, Ampofo K, Stockmann C, et al. Community surveillance of respiratory viruses among families in the Utah better identification of germs-longitudinal viral epidemiology (BIG-LoVE) study. Clin Infect Dis 2015;61(8):1217–24.
38. Martin ET, Kuypers J, McRoberts JP, et al. Human bocavirus 1 primary infection and shedding in infants. J Infect Dis 2015;212(4):516–24.
39. Jartti T, Hedman K, Jartti L, et al. Human bocavirus-the first 5 years. Rev Med Virol 2012;22(1):46–64.

40. Schildgen O, Muller A, Allander T, et al. Human bocavirus: passenger or pathogen in acute respiratory tract infections? Clin Microbiol Rev 2008;21(2): 291–304, table of contents.

41. Guido M, Tumolo MR, Verri T, et al. Human bocavirus: current knowledge and future challenges. World J Gastroenterol 2016;22(39):8684–97.

42. Lukkarinen H, Soderlund-Venermo M, Vuorinen T, et al. Human bocavirus 1 may suppress rhinovirus-associated immune response in wheezing children. J Allergy Clin Immunol 2014;133(1):256–8.e1-4.

43. Del Rosal T, Garcia-Garcia ML, Calvo C, et al. Recurrent wheezing and asthma after bocavirus bronchiolitis. Allergol Immunopathol (Madr) 2016;44(5):410–4.

44. Molinari NA, Ortega-Sanchez IR, Messonnier ML, et al. The annual impact of seasonal influenza in the US: measuring disease burden and costs. Vaccine 2007; 25(27):5086–96.

45. Khetsuriani N, Kazerouni NN, Erdman DD, et al. Prevalence of viral respiratory tract infections in children with asthma. J Allergy Clin Immunol 2007;119(2): 314–21.

46. Tan WC, Xiang X, Qiu D, et al. Epidemiology of respiratory viruses in patients hospitalized with near-fatal asthma, acute exacerbations of asthma, or chronic obstructive pulmonary disease. Am J Med 2003;115(4):272–7.

47. Teichtahl H, Buckmaster N, Pertnikovs E. The incidence of respiratory tract infection in adults requiring hospitalization for asthma. Chest 1997;112(3):591–6.

48. Shim DH, Park YA, Kim MJ, et al. Pandemic influenza virus, pH1N1, induces asthmatic symptoms via activation of innate lymphoid cells. Pediatr Allergy Immunol 2015;26(8):780–8.

49. Ravanetti L, Dijkhuis A, Dekker T, et al. IL-33 drives influenza-induced asthma exacerbations by halting innate and adaptive antiviral immunity. J Allergy Clin Immunol 2019;143(4):1355–70.

50. Ravanetti L, Dijkhuis A, Sabogal Pineros YS, et al. An early innate response underlies severe influenza-induced exacerbations of asthma in a novel steroid-insensitive and anti-IL-5-responsive mouse model. Allergy 2017;72(5):737–53.

51. Lund S, Walford HH, Doherty TA. Type 2 innate lymphoid cells in allergic disease. Curr Immunol Rev 2013;9(4):214–21.

52. Chang YJ, Kim HY, Albacker LA, et al. Innate lymphoid cells mediate influenza-induced airway hyper-reactivity independently of adaptive immunity. Nat Immunol 2011;12(7):631–8.

53. Contoli M, Message SD, Laza-Stanca V, et al. Role of deficient type III interferon-lambda production in asthma exacerbations. Nat Med 2006;12(9):1023–6.

54. Forbes RL, Gibson PG, Murphy VE, et al. Impaired type I and III interferon response to rhinovirus infection during pregnancy and asthma. Thorax 2012; 67(3):209–14.

55. Sykes A, Macintyre J, Edwards MR, et al. Rhinovirus-induced interferon production is not deficient in well controlled asthma. Thorax 2014;69(3):240–6.

56. Patel DA, You Y, Huang G, et al. Interferon response and respiratory virus control are preserved in bronchial epithelial cells in asthma. J Allergy Clin Immunol 2014; 134(6):1402–12.e7.

57. Kloepfer KM, Olenec JP, Lee WM, et al. Increased H1N1 infection rate in children with asthma. Am J Respir Crit Care Med 2012;185(12):1275–9.

58. Grohskopf LA, Sokolow LZ, Broder KR, et al. Prevention and control of seasonal influenza with vaccines: recommendations of the advisory committee on immunization practices-United States, 2018-19 influenza season. MMWR Recomm Rep 2018;67(3):1–20.

59. Cullen G, Martin J, O'Donnell J, et al. Surveillance of the first 205 confirmed hospitalised cases of pandemic H1N1 influenza in Ireland, 28 April - 3 October 2009. Euro Surveill 2009;14(44) [pii:19389].
60. Santillan Salas CF, Mehra S, Pardo Crespo MR, et al. Asthma and severity of 2009 novel H1N1 influenza: a population-based case-control study. J Asthma 2013; 50(10):1069–76.
61. Veerapandian R, Snyder JD, Samarasinghe AE. Influenza in asthmatics: for better or for worse? Front Immunol 2018;9:1843.
62. Van Kerkhove MD, Vandemaele KA, Shinde V, et al. Risk factors for severe outcomes following 2009 influenza A (H1N1) infection: a global pooled analysis. PLoS Med 2011;8(7):e1001053.
63. Louie JK, Acosta M, Winter K, et al. Factors associated with death or hospitalization due to pandemic 2009 influenza A(H1N1) infection in California. JAMA 2009; 302(17):1896–902.
64. Myles PR, Semple MG, Lim WS, et al. Predictors of clinical outcome in a national hospitalised cohort across both waves of the influenza A/H1N1 pandemic 2009-2010 in the UK. Thorax 2012;67(8):709–17.
65. Myles P, Nguyen-Van-Tam JS, Semple MG, et al. Differences between asthmatics and nonasthmatics hospitalised with influenza A infection. Eur Respir J 2013; 41(4):824–31.
66. Samarasinghe AE, Melo RC, Duan S, et al. Eosinophils promote antiviral immunity in mice infected with influenza A virus. J Immunol 2017;198(8):3214–26.
67. An S, Jeon YJ, Jo A, et al. Initial influenza virus replication can be limited in allergic asthma through rapid induction of type III interferons in respiratory epithelium. Front Immunol 2018;9:986.
68. Ishikawa H, Sasaki H, Fukui T, et al. Mice with asthma are more resistant to influenza virus infection and NK cells activated by the induction of asthma have potentially protective effects. J Clin Immunol 2012;32(2):256–67.
69. Cates CJ, Rowe BH. Vaccines for preventing influenza in people with asthma. Cochrane Database Syst Rev 2013;(2):CD000364.
70. Nicholson KG, Nguyen-Van-Tam JS, Ahmed AH, et al. Randomised placebo-controlled crossover trial on effect of inactivated influenza vaccine on pulmonary function in asthma. Lancet 1998;351(9099):326–31.
71. Bueving HJ, Bernsen RM, de Jongste JC, et al. Does influenza vaccination exacerbate asthma in children? Vaccine 2004;23(1):91–6.
72. The American Lung Association Asthma Clinical Research Centers. The safety of inactivated influenza vaccine in adults and children with asthma. N Engl J Med 2001;345(21):1529–36.
73. Turner PJ, Southern J, Andrews NJ, et al. Safety of live attenuated influenza vaccine in atopic children with egg allergy. J Allergy Clin Immunol 2015;136(2): 376–81.

Sinus Infections, Inflammation, and Asthma

Anna G. Staudacher, MS, Whitney W. Stevens, MD, PhD*

KEYWORDS

- Acute rhinosinusitis • Chronic rhinosinusitis • Nasal polyp • Infection • Inflammation
- Asthma • Microbiome

KEY POINTS

- Rhinosinusitis is clinically defined as the presence of nasal drainage (anterior or posterior), nasal congestion, facial pain/pressure, and/or reduced sense of smell.
- In acute rhinosinusitis, nasal symptoms last for less than 12 weeks and inflammation is often secondary to a viral or bacterial infection.
- In chronic rhinosinusitis (CRS), nasal symptoms persist for longer than 12 weeks and the inflammation observed is secondary to impairments in the epithelial barrier, dysregulation of the host immune response, and potentially infections (or colonization) by pathogens.
- CRS and asthma have a strong clinical association and share similar pathophysiologic mechanisms in support of the unified airway hypothesis.

INTRODUCTION

The unified airway hypothesis suggests that the nose and lungs are not separate organ systems but instead are part of the same continuum. Inflammation of the upper respiratory tract can affect the lower respiratory tract and vice versa. Viral and bacterial respiratory pathogens have long been known to induce acute inflammation in the airways and some have been implicated in the development of more chronic diseases. Rhinosinusitis and asthma are 2 common respiratory diseases that have been linked together on a clinical, as well as a pathophysiologic, basis (**Fig. 1**). In this review, associations between rhinosinusitis and asthma will be explored, with particular emphasis placed on the role of infections and inflammation.

Disclosure Statements: A.G. Staudacher and W.W. Stevens have no financial disclosures.
Division of Allergy and Immunology, Department of Medicine, Northwestern University Feinberg School of Medicine, 211 East Ontario Street Suite 1000, Chicago, IL 60611, USA
* Corresponding author.
E-mail address: whitney-stevens@northwestern.edu

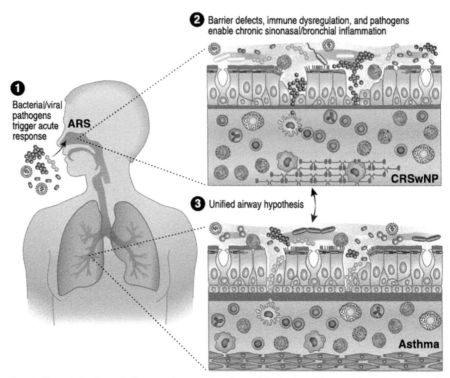

Fig. 1. Sinus infections, inflammation, and asthma. (1) Viral and bacterial respiratory pathogens are the most common cause of ARS, can exacerbate preexisting asthma, and potentially can lead to the development of asthma in certain populations. (2) In chronic rhinosinusitis with nasal polyp (CRSwNP) and asthma, impaired tight junctions, dysregulated immune responses, and possible infections (or colonization) by pathogens contribute to chronic airway inflammation. (3) The unified airway hypothesis suggests that upper airway inflammation can influence lower airway disease and vice versa further supporting the strong clinical association noted between CRSwNP and asthma. (*Courtesy of* J. Schaffer, MAMS, Chicago, IL.)

ACUTE RHINOSINUSITIS

Acute rhinosinusitis (ARS) is defined as the presence of nasal drainage (anterior or posterior), nasal congestion, facial pain/pressure, and/or reduced sense of smell. Depending on which guidelines are followed, ARS symptoms last either for less than 4 weeks[1] or 12 weeks.[2,3] ARS is a clinical diagnosis, and objective confirmation by sinus computed tomography (CT) scan or nasal endoscopy is generally not indicated. Patients can have more than one episode of ARS each year but importantly, they are asymptomatic in the intervening periods.

Acute rhinosinusitis is extremely common. Studies specifying ARS found a disease prevalence of 6% to 15%,[2,4] with an estimated 0.035% of the population suffering from recurrent episodes.[5] Between 2006 and 2010, there were an estimated 21.4 million ambulatory care visits with a primary diagnosis of ARS.[6] Furthermore, in 2015 alone, acute upper respiratory infection (or presumed ARS) was one of the top 20 leading diagnoses for outpatient office visits.[7]

PATHOGENS AND ACUTE RHINOSINUSITIS

Certain individuals may be predisposed to rhinosinusitis due to allergic rhinitis, allergy, smoking history, or a mechanical obstruction of the sinus ostium.[2,3] However, for most patients, upper respiratory tract infections are most often responsible. ARS is classically divided into 2 main subtypes based on the cause and duration of symptoms. Acute viral sinusitis lasts for less than 10 days with a rapid peak and then decline in nasal symptoms. The most common viruses isolated in ARS are rhinoviruses and coronaviruses, but respiratory syncytial virus (RSV), influenza virus, parainfluenza virus, enterovirus, and adenovirus can also be the causes.

If acute upper respiratory symptoms persist for greater than 10 days, or if symptoms initially improve but then worsen again, acute bacterial rhinosinusitis (ABRS) should be considered. In these patients, additional symptoms that are more likely to be observed include persistent purulent nasal drainage, severe facial pain, fever, and dental pain.[1–3] ABRS generally develops following acute viral rhinosinusitis but overall is not a common occurrence, developing in only 0.5% to 2% of cases.[8,9]

Pathogens most associated with acute bacterial rhinosinusitis include *Streptococcus pneumoniae, Haemophilus influenzae, Moraxella catarrhalis, Staphylococcus aureus*, and *Streptococcus pyogenes*. Since the introduction of the Pneumococcal conjugate vaccine, the pathogen profile of ARS has changed with a declining incidence of *S pneumoniae* and increasing incidence of *H influenzae, S pyogenes*, and *S aureus*.[10] Anaerobes such as Fusobacterium, Peptostreptococcus, and Bacteroides spp. account for a smaller percentage of ABRS cases.[11,12] Infections with gram-negative bacteria are unusual in community settings and the presence of Enterobacteriaceae or Pseudomonas spp. suggest a chronic underlying condition or a dental infection that has migrated to the sinuses.[13,14]

ACUTE RHINOSINUSITIS AND ASTHMA

It is well known that acute upper respiratory infections are capable of exacerbating preexisting asthma. However, one episode of ARS is not generally associated with having a higher risk of developing asthma per se. As discussed earlier and in the preceding chapters, there are specific pathogens associated with ARS that have also been associated with the development asthma. For example, RSV infections in infancy are a risk factor for developing allergic asthma in adolescence.[15–17] Likewise, human rhinovirus in infants was also associated with higher incidence of having asthma as an adult.[18–21] Elucidating the key mechanistic links between specific viral (or bacterial) pathogens and development of new onset asthma is critical not only for better understanding of the link between the upper and lower respiratory tract but also for identifying potentially modifiable factors that could lead to disease prevention.

CHRONIC RHINOSINUSITIS

In contrast to ARS, chronic rhinosinusitis (CRS) is characterized by chronic inflammation of the sinonasal mucosa. The diagnosis of CRS is made clinically in patients exhibiting anterior or posterior nasal drainage, nasal congestion, facial pain or pressure, and/or decreased sense of smell for greater than 12 weeks.[2] Among patients reporting CRS symptoms, objective evidence of chronic inflammation should be confirmed either by direct visualization with nasal endoscopy or by sinus CT scan. A small subset of patients with CRS (~20%) also has nasal polyps, which are benign inflammatory outgrowths of the sinonasal mucosa.[2,22] Such patients are aptly referred to as having CRS with nasal polyps (CRSwNP) leaving the remaining majority of patients with CRS as having CRS without nasal polyps (CRSsNP).

Using symptom-based criteria, the overall prevalence of CRS within a primary care US population was 11.9%.[23] This is similar to earlier studies in Europe that reported the prevalence of CRS to be 10.9%.[24] Among tertiary care populations, however, the prevalence of CRS is estimated to be even higher given a possible referral bias. In a longitudinal study of adults reporting CRS symptoms in a US general population, the lifetime prevalence of CRS was estimated to be 27.5% with an annual cumulative incidence of almost 2%.[25] As a comparison, the lifetime prevalence of asthma in adults was 13.9% according to the 2016 National Health Interview Survey.[7] The annual cost of these diseases has been estimated to be between $22 to $33 billion for CRS[26–28] and $81.9 billion for asthma.[29] Taken together, asthma and CRS are prevalent within the US population and can place large socioeconomic and financial burdens on affected patients and the health care system.

CHRONIC RHINOSINUSITIS AND ASTHMA: CLINICAL OBSERVATIONS

The relationship between CRS and asthma remains of great interest from both a clinical as well as a pathophysiologic perspective. Although not every patient with CRS has asthma and vice versa, a strong and independent association between these conditions has been reported. In a large European study, asthma was more prevalent in patients with CRS than without (odds ratio [OR] 2.71).[30] Furthermore, patients with CRSwNP were more likely to have asthma than those with CRSsNP,[31] with one study reporting asthma in as many as 48.3% of patients with CRSwNP compared with only 16.5% with CRSsNP.[32] A study from France also found that most of the asthmatics had abnormal sinus CT scans.[33] Similarly, asthmatic patients with CRS were more likely to have nasal polyps than nonasthmatic patients with CRS.[34]

Exactly when (and why) patients develop CRS and asthma remains unclear. CRS is primarily a disease of adulthood, and given that the sinuses do not entirely form until late adolescence, other diseases, including cystic fibrosis, should first be considered in children presenting with nasal polyps.[35] Although asthma can develop either in childhood or later in life, CRS is more significantly linked with adult-onset asthma.[30] In particular, patients with CRS were more likely to develop nasal polyps if they had adult-onset versus childhood-onset disease.[36] Asthma may precede the diagnosis of CRSwNP[37] or develop following the diagnosis of CRSsNP.[38] However, it is more likely that the time frame in which CRS and asthma develop is variable and depends on a variety of yet to be identified factors.

The association between CRS and asthma has important clinical implications. Among 250 patients with CRS at a tertiary care facility, those with asthma had significantly worse sinus CT and nasal endoscopic scores compared with patients with CRS without asthma.[31,39] Furthermore, the more severe the asthma, the greater the likelihood of having severe CRS.[40] In the United States, the Severe Asthma Research Program identified distinct clinical phenotypes of severe asthma, with the cluster of asthmatics with the most severe airflow limitations at baseline being the same group with the highest percentage of reported sinus disease.[41]

Although asthma can influence sinonasal disease severity, CRS is also associated with more severe asthma. Patients with both CRS and asthma had lower lung function (percentage predicted forced expiratory volume in the first second of expiration and forced vital capacity) and quality of life when compared with patients with asthma alone.[42] Furthermore, severe CRS is an independent risk factor for having frequent asthma exacerbations (OR 5.5),[43] and patients with severe asthma were more likely to undergo sinus surgery for nasal polyps when compared with patients with mild asthma.[44] Finally, when compared with patients with CRSwNP alone, those with both CRSwNP and asthma were significantly more likely to have enhanced sinonasal disease on sinus CT scan, to undergo more sinus surgeries and to be dependent on chronic oral corticosteroids for management of their disease.[45] Taken together, these studies highlight the fact that CRS and asthma are frequently associated together in the clinical setting and the presence of one can significantly enhance the severity of the other. As such, it remains important to evaluate patients with CRS for asthma as well as asthmatic patients for CRS to optimize disease diagnosis and management.

CHRONIC RHINOSINUSITIS AND ASTHMA: PATHOPHYSIOLOGIC OBSERVATIONS

To better understand the mechanisms contributing to the clinical associations observed between CRS and asthma, nasal and pulmonary tissues would ideally be isolated at the same time from the same patient and then compared. Not surprisingly, such studies are exceedingly rare but in one such investigation a strong correlation in inflammatory profiles was observed between nasal polyp and bronchial biopsies.[46] Larger mechanistic studies have also separately advanced the knowledge of the underlying cellular and molecular processes contributing to either asthma or CRS pathogenesis.[47–49] Although an exhaustive summary of these findings is beyond the scope of the current review, focus will be placed on highlighting some of the key features of CRS especially in comparison to asthma.

As mentioned previously, the strongest association between asthma and CRS is observed among patients with CRSwNP. This is not surprising because, similar to what is observed in most of the asthmatics, nasal polyps in the United States and Europe are predominantly characterized by type 2 inflammation.[50–53] Eosinophils as well as their granule proteins (eg, eosinophil cationic protein, eosinophil peroxidase) are elevated in nasal polyps compared with healthy control sinonasal tissue.[50,54,55] Other type 2 immune cells, including mast cells, basophils, and group 2 innate lymphoid cells, are also increased in nasal polyps.[56–61] This robust type 2 inflammatory response is orchestrated in part by elevated levels of prosurvival and chemotactic mediators such as interleukin 4 (IL-4), IL-5, IL-13, eotaxins, and thymic stromal lymphopoietin.[55,62–64]

In contrast to CRSwNP, CRSsNP was originally characterized by type 1 inflammation due to elevated levels of interferon gamma (IFNγ) detected in this subtype.[54,63] However, subsequent studies have challenged this dichotomy and shown no differences in IFNγ levels observed between CRS subtypes.[50,55,65] A more recent comprehensive analysis evaluating the expression of several inflammatory mediators in different sinonasal tissues in CRS suggested that CRSsNP is instead a heterogenous disease.[66] In this work, 23% of patients with CRSsNP had a predominant type 1 phenotype as assessed by IFNγ gene expression levels above the 95th percentile of what was observed in healthy controls. Furthermore, 36% of patients with CRSsNP had increased gene expression of type 2 inflammatory mediators above the 95th percentile of what was measured in controls.[66] The clinical relevance of these different endotypes, and why CRSsNP in general has a weaker association with asthma compared with CRSwNP, is unclear and remains the focus of ongoing investigations.

The adaptive immune response has also been characterized in CRS with both T and B cells thought to play important roles. T cells that produce type 2 inflammatory cytokines are increased in nasal polyps.[50,67] In addition, naïve B cells and plasma cells are elevated in nasal polyps when compared with healthy controls.[68–70] Total levels of antibodies (including immunoglobulin E [IgE] and IgG) are significantly higher in nasal polyps when compared with peripheral blood of matched patients as well as healthy sinonasal tissue.[69] The function of this local antibody production as well as the specificity of the antibodies generated is still largely unknown. However, IgG antibodies that are self-reactive[71] and IgE antibodies against *S aureus* and its enterotoxins[72] as well as other bacteria such as *H influenzae*[73] have been described.

Besides having an enhanced immunologic response, CRS is also characterized by a dysfunctional epithelial barrier with tight junctions, host defense proteins, and mucociliary clearance factors all found to be impaired.[47,74,75] These findings, in most regard, are similar to what has been reported in the lower respiratory tract of asthma.[76,77] A weakened epithelial barrier can have profound consequences, because the upper and lower respiratory tracts are constantly exposed to millions of microbes daily. In a healthy host, these microbes are routinely cleared without inciting an inflammatory response, but in CRS such processes are impaired.[78] It remains unknown if the impaired epithelial barrier leads to increased pathogen recognition by the host or if the exposure to pathogens in the respiratory tract leads to epithelial barrier damage. Either way, the endpoint could be the initiation and potentiation of a robust immunologic response.

PATHOGENS AND CHRONIC RHINOSINUSITIS

S aureus is known to colonize the nasal mucosa,[79] and it has been one of the most studied microbes in CRS. One hypothesis suggests that the bacteria itself is directly involved in driving CRS pathogenesis, damaging the epithelial barrier and activating the host immune response. Ex vivo studies of nasal polyp explants infected with *S aureus* showed reduced gene expression levels of various tight junction proteins when compared with similarly infected healthy nasal mucosa.[80] In addition, in a separate study, *S aureus* was reported to bind to TLR2 and induce type 2 cytokine release from cultured epithelial cells.[81] This in turn could potentially explain how colonization with *S aureus* in the nasal cavity could lead to the development of a chronic immunologic response. However, what is not addressed in these studies is why only some patients who are colonized with *S aureus* go on to develop CRS. Furthermore, in patients with CRSwNP, the presence of *S aureus* was associated with more severe sinus inflammation on CT scans but not sinonasal symptoms, suggesting this pathogen alone is not fully responsible for all aspects of disease.[82]

Another hypothesis is that the immune response to *S aureus* is important in CRS pathogenesis. In support of this, type 2 inflammatory mediators were significantly elevated in nasal polyps of patients with detectable levels of specific IgE antibodies to *S aureus* enterotoxins (SAE), but no correlation was found between these markers and the presence of *S aureus* in the tissue.[83] Specific antibodies to SAEs can induce basophil degranulation[72] and mast cell activation,[84,85] providing another possible mechanism by which *S aureus* could contribute to chronic type 2 inflammation. However, in a separate study, although patients with CRSwNP were more likely to have elevated serum levels of specific IgE to SAE compared with healthy controls, there was no association between these antibody levels and sinus disease severity as assessed by CT scan.[86]

It is important to note that not all patients with CRS are colonized with *S aureus*, with one study reporting colonization rates of 27.3% in CRS versus 33.3% in healthy controls.[87] Likewise, only 27.8% of patients who were colonized with *S aureus* had detectable specific IgE to SAE.[87] However, both colonization with *S aureus* and the presence of specific IgE to SAE were significantly higher in those patients who had both CRSwNP and asthma (66.7% and 53.8%, respectively).[87] In a meta-analysis, nasal

S aureus colonization was only modestly associated with asthma prevalence (OR 1.19) in the general population or, after adjusting for study bias, among a subset of patients with CRS (OR 1.21).[88] However, patients with detectable specific IgE to SAE were more likely to have severe asthma[89–91] as well as reduced lung function and increased airway reversibility to bronchodilation.[92] Taken together, specific IgE to SAE and/or *S aureus* may be important in CRS pathogenesis and related to comorbid asthma in a select group of patients, but the exact mechanisms for these associations are still unclear.

In addition to *S aureus*, other bacteria including coagulase-negative staphylococci, *H influenzae, S pneumoniae, Moraxella catarrhalis, Corynebacterium* spp., and *Propionibacterium acnes* have been detected in sinonasal samples of patients with CRS either by nasal culture or by measuring bacteria-specific 16S ribosomal DNA.[93–97] Total bacterial counts did not correlate with sinus disease severity[98] but, when compared with healthy controls, one study found patients with CRS to have significantly lower Actinobacteria levels (and lower *Corynebacterium* spp.) as well as reduced relative abundance of the genus *Peptoniphilus*.[99]

Differences have also been reported in the nasal microbiome in patients with CRS with or without asthma. In one study, those with asthma had increased abundance of the phylum Proteobacteria, *M catarrhalis*, and *Staphylococcus xylosus* and decreased abundance of genus *Corynebacterium, Geobacter anodireducens/sulfurreducens*, and *Pelomonas puraquae*.[100] In a separate study of 111 CRS cases, no significant difference in the diversity of bacterial species was noted between patients with CRS with and without asthma.[101] Although, the relative abundance of *Streptococcus* spp. was significantly higher in patients with CRS with asthma as compared with without.[101] Furthermore, asthmatic patients with CRS with emergency room (ER) visits for asthma had significantly higher relative abundance of Proteobacteria phylum (likely due to increased *Burkholderia spp.*) than patients who did not visit the ER for symptoms.[101] These findings are interesting given that *Streptococcus* has been linked to asthma development in children[102] and *Burkholderia* is associated with decreased lung function in patients with cystic fibrosis.[103] However, how these bacteria are specifically involved in CRS pathogenesis is not known.

By comparing the frequency, abundance, and diversity of bacteria in patients with CRS with that observed in healthy controls, the ideal goal would be to identify particular bacteria that could be protective against or predispose toward developing the disease. Unfortunately, most studies to date have been descriptive without causality shown. In addition, there are significant variations between studies with differences in the patient demographics, where within the sinonasal cavity samples were collected, how the data were generated, and the methods by which the data were analyzed. To date, no one particular pathogen has been implicated in CRS, but an overall increased abundance and decreased diversity of the microbiome has been observed.[104,105] It is thus likely that differences in the microbiome are important in CRS pathogenesis and in the link between CRS and asthma. However, further studies are needed to investigate what these key factors could be.

FUTURE CONSIDERATIONS/SUMMARY

There is a strong and important relationship between the upper and lower respiratory tracts whereby inflammation in one environment can influence the other. In acute rhinosinusitis, exposures to viral and bacterial pathogens are the primary driver for acute inflammation in the nose, which can then lead to exacerbations of asthma. In contrast, it remains unclear what precise role infections (or colonization) in the airways play in the development of CRS, but other factors, including the presence of an impaired epithelial barrier and dysregulated immune responses, can promote the chronic inflammation that is observed in CRS. Clinically, CRS is strongly associated with asthma with both diseases sharing similar underlying inflammatory processes. In conclusion, significant advancements have been made in identifying sinus infections and inflammation as important in asthma pathogenesis, but additional work is needed to further define the specific mechanisms responsible for connecting the nose with the lungs.

REFERENCES

1. Rosenfeld RM, Piccirillo JF, Chandrasekhar SS, et al. Clinical practice guideline (update): adult sinusitis executive summary. Otolaryngol Head Neck Surg 2015; 152:598–609.
2. Fokkens WJ, Lund VJ, Mullol J, et al. European Position Paper on Rhinosinusitis and Nasal Polyps 2012. Rhinol Suppl 2012; 23:p. 3. preceding table of contents, 1-298.
3. Peters AT, Spector S, Hsu J, et al. Diagnosis and management of rhinosinusitis: a practice parameter update. Ann Allergy Asthma Immunol 2014;113:347–85.
4. Bhattacharyya N. Contemporary assessment of the disease burden of sinusitis. Am J Rhinol Allergy 2009;23:392–5.
5. Bhattacharyya N, Grebner J, Martinson NG. Recurrent acute rhinosinusitis: epidemiology and health care cost burden. Otolaryngol Head Neck Surg 2012;146:307–12.
6. Smith SS, Evans CT, Tan BK, et al. National burden of antibiotic use for adult rhinosinusitis. J Allergy Clin Immunol 2013;132:1230–2.
7. NCHS. National Ambulatory Medical Care Survey. 2015. Available at: https://www.cdc.gov/nchs/data/ahcd/namcs_summary/2015_namcs_web_tables.pdf. Accessed April 11, 2019.
8. Gwaltney JM Jr. Acute community-acquired sinusitis. Clin Infect Dis 1996;23: 1209–23.
9. Piccirillo JF. Clinical practice. Acute bacterial sinusitis. N Engl J Med 2004;351: 902–10.
10. Brook I, Gober AE. Frequency of recovery of pathogens from the nasopharynx of children with acute maxillary sinusitis before and after the introduction of vaccination with the 7-valent pneumococcal vaccine. Int J Pediatr Otorhinolaryngol 2007;71:575–9.
11. Brook I. Bacteriology of acute and chronic frontal sinusitis. Arch Otolaryngol Head Neck Surg 2002;128:583–5.
12. Brook I. The role of anaerobic bacteria in sinusitis. Anaerobe 2006;12:5–12.
13. Brook I. Microbiology of intracranial abscesses associated with sinusitis of odontogenic origin. Ann Otol Rhinol Laryngol 2006;115:917–20.
14. Brook I. Sinusitis of odontogenic origin. Otolaryngol Head Neck Surg 2006;135: 349–55.
15. Wu P, Dupont WD, Griffin MR, et al. Evidence of a causal role of winter virus infection during infancy in early childhood asthma. Am J Respir Crit Care Med 2008;178:1123–9.
16. Sigurs N, Gustafsson PM, Bjarnason R, et al. Severe respiratory syncytial virus bronchiolitis in infancy and asthma and allergy at age 13. Am J Respir Crit Care Med 2005;171:137–41.

17. Feldman AS, He Y, Moore ML, et al. Toward primary prevention of asthma. Reviewing the evidence for early-life respiratory viral infections as modifiable risk factors to prevent childhood asthma. Am J Respir Crit Care Med 2015;191: 34–44.

18. Jackson DJ, Gangnon RE, Evans MD, et al. Wheezing rhinovirus illnesses in early life predict asthma development in high-risk children. Am J Respir Crit Care Med 2008;178:667–72.

19. Lemanske RF Jr, Jackson DJ, Gangnon RE, et al. Rhinovirus illnesses during infancy predict subsequent childhood wheezing. J Allergy Clin Immunol 2005; 116:571–7.

20. Busse WW, Lemanske RF Jr, Gern JE. Role of viral respiratory infections in asthma and asthma exacerbations. Lancet 2010;376:826–34.

21. Soto-Quiros M, Avila L, Platts-Mills TA, et al. High titers of IgE antibody to dust mite allergen and risk for wheezing among asthmatic children infected with rhinovirus. J Allergy Clin Immunol 2012;129:1499–505.

22. Orlandi RR, Kingdom TT, Hwang PH. International consensus statement on allergy and rhinology: rhinosinusitis executive summary. Int Forum Allergy Rhinol 2016;6(Suppl 1):S3–21.

23. Hirsch AG, Stewart WF, Sundaresan AS, et al. Nasal and sinus symptoms and chronic rhinosinusitis in a population-based sample. Allergy 2017;72:274–81.

24. Hastan D, Fokkens WJ, Bachert C, et al. Chronic rhinosinusitis in Europe–an underestimated disease. A GA(2)LEN study. Allergy 2011;66:1216–23.

25. Sundaresan AS, Hirsch AG, Young AJ, et al. Longitudinal evaluation of chronic rhinosinusitis symptoms in a population-based sample. J Allergy Clin Immunol Pract 2018;6:1327–35.

26. Bhattacharyya N, Orlandi RR, Grebner J, et al. Cost burden of chronic rhinosinusitis: a claims-based study. Otolaryngol Head Neck Surg 2011;144:440–5.

27. Rudmik L. Economics of chronic rhinosinusitis. Curr Allergy Asthma Rep 2017; 17:20.

28. Smith KA, Orlandi RR, Rudmik L. Cost of adult chronic rhinosinusitis: a systematic review. Laryngoscope 2015;125:1547–56.

29. Nurmagambetov T, Kuwahara R, Garbe P. The economic burden of asthma in the United States, 2008-2013. Ann Am Thorac Soc 2018;15:348–56.

30. Jarvis D, Newson R, Lotvall J, et al. Asthma in adults and its association with chronic rhinosinusitis: the GA2LEN survey in Europe. Allergy 2012;67:91–8.

31. Batra PS, Tong L, Citardi MJ. Analysis of comorbidities and objective parameters in refractory chronic rhinosinusitis. Laryngoscope 2013;123(Suppl 7): S1–11.

32. Promsopa C, Kansara S, Citardi MJ, et al. Prevalence of confirmed asthma varies in chronic rhinosinusitis subtypes. Int Forum Allergy Rhinol 2016;6:373–7.

33. Bresciani M, Paradis L, Des Roches A, et al. Rhinosinusitis in severe asthma. J Allergy Clin Immunol 2001;107:73–80.

34. Pearlman AN, Chandra RK, Chang D, et al. Relationships between severity of chronic rhinosinusitis and nasal polyposis, asthma, and atopy. Am J Rhinol Allergy 2009;23:145–8.

35. Hamilos DL. Chronic rhinosinusitis in patients with cystic fibrosis. J Allergy Clin Immunol Pract 2016;4:605–12.

36. Staniorski CJ, Price CPE, Weibman AR, et al. Asthma onset pattern and patient outcomes in a chronic rhinosinusitis population. Int Forum Allergy Rhinol 2018;8: 495–503.

37. Tan BK, Chandra RK, Pollak J, et al. Incidence and associated premorbid diagnoses of patients with chronic rhinosinusitis. J Allergy Clin Immunol 2013;131: 1350–60.

38. Hirsch AG, Yan XS, Sundaresan AS, et al. Five-year risk of incident disease following a diagnosis of chronic rhinosinusitis. Allergy 2015;70:1613–21.

39. ten Brinke A, Grootendorst DC, Schmidt JT, et al. Chronic sinusitis in severe asthma is related to sputum eosinophilia. J Allergy Clin Immunol 2002;109: 621–6.

40. Lin DC, Chandra RK, Tan BK, et al. Association between severity of asthma and degree of chronic rhinosinusitis. Am J Rhinol Allergy 2011;25:205–8.

41. Moore WC, Meyers DA, Wenzel SE, et al. Identification of asthma phenotypes using cluster analysis in the Severe Asthma Research Program. Am J Respir Crit Care Med 2010;181:315–23.

42. Ek A, Middelveld RJ, Bertilsson H, et al. Chronic rhinosinusitis in asthma is a negative predictor of quality of life: results from the Swedish GA(2)LEN survey. Allergy 2013;68:1314–21.

43. ten Brinke A, Sterk PJ, Masclee AA, et al. Risk factors of frequent exacerbations in difficult-to-treat asthma. Eur Respir J 2005;26:812–8.

44. Wu W, Bleecker E, Moore W, et al. Unsupervised phenotyping of Severe Asthma Research Program participants using expanded lung data. J Allergy Clin Immunol 2014;133:1280–8.

45. Stevens WW, Peters AT, Hirsch AG, et al. Clinical characteristics of patients with chronic rhinosinusitis with nasal polyps, asthma, and aspirin-exacerbated respiratory disease. J Allergy Clin Immunol Pract 2017;5:1061–70.

46. Hakansson K, Bachert C, Konge L, et al. Airway inflammation in chronic rhinosinusitis with nasal polyps and asthma: the united airways concept further supported. PLoS One 2015;10:e0127228.

47. Schleimer RP. Immunopathogenesis of chronic rhinosinusitis and nasal polyposis. Annu Rev Pathol 2017;12:331–57.

48. Holgate ST, Wenzel S, Postma DS, et al. Asthma. Nat Rev Dis Primers 2015;1: 15025.

49. Ray A, Raundhal M, Oriss TB, et al. Current concepts of severe asthma. J Clin Invest 2016;126:2394–403.

50. Zhang N, Van Zele T, Perez-Novo C, et al. Different types of T-effector cells orchestrate mucosal inflammation in chronic sinus disease. J Allergy Clin Immunol 2008;122:961–8.

51. Wang X, Zhang N, Bo M, et al. Diversity of TH cytokine profiles in patients with chronic rhinosinusitis: a multicenter study in Europe, Asia, and Oceania. J Allergy Clin Immunol 2016;138:1344–53.

52. Caminati M, Pham DL, Bagnasco D, et al. Type 2 immunity in asthma. World Allergy Organ J 2018;11:13.

53. Kubo M. Innate and adaptive type 2 immunity in lung allergic inflammation. Immunol Rev 2017;278:162–72.

54. Van Zele T, Claeys S, Gevaert P, et al. Differentiation of chronic sinus diseases by measurement of inflammatory mediators. Allergy 2006;61:1280–9.

55. Stevens WW, Ocampo CJ, Berdnikovs S, et al. Cytokines in chronic rhinosinusitis. role in eosinophilia and aspirin-exacerbated respiratory disease. Am J Respir Crit Care Med 2015;192:682–94.

56. Shaw JL, Ashoori F, Fakhri S, et al. Increased percentage of mast cells within sinonasal mucosa of chronic rhinosinusitis with nasal polyp patients independent of atopy. Int Forum Allergy Rhinol 2012;2:233–40.

57. Takabayashi T, Kato A, Peters AT, et al. Glandular mast cells with distinct phenotype are highly elevated in chronic rhinosinusitis with nasal polyps. J Allergy Clin Immunol 2012;130:410–20.
58. Kagoya R, Kondo K, Baba S, et al. Correlation of basophil infiltration in nasal polyps with the severity of chronic rhinosinusitis. Ann Allergy Asthma Immunol 2015;114:30–5.
59. Mahdavinia M, Carter RG, Ocampo CJ, et al. Basophils are elevated in nasal polyps of patients with chronic rhinosinusitis without aspirin sensitivity. J Allergy Clin Immunol 2014;133:1759–63.
60. Poposki JA, Klingler AI, Tan BK, et al. Group 2 innate lymphoid cells are elevated and activated in chronic rhinosinusitis with nasal polyps. Immun Inflamm Dis 2017;5:233–43.
61. Shaw JL, Fakhri S, Citardi MJ, et al. IL-33-responsive innate lymphoid cells are an important source of IL-13 in chronic rhinosinusitis with nasal polyps. Am J Respir Crit Care Med 2013;188:432–9.
62. Hulse KE, Stevens WW, Tan BK, et al. Pathogenesis of nasal polyposis. Clin Exp Allergy 2015;45:328–46.
63. Van Bruaene N, Perez-Novo CA, Basinski TM, et al. T-cell regulation in chronic paranasal sinus disease. J Allergy Clin Immunol 2008;121:1435–41, 41.
64. Nagarkar DR, Poposki JA, Tan BK, et al. Thymic stromal lymphopoietin activity is increased in nasal polyps of patients with chronic rhinosinusitis. J Allergy Clin Immunol 2013;132:593–600.
65. Van Bruaene N, C PN, Van Crombruggen K, et al. Inflammation and remodelling patterns in early stage chronic rhinosinusitis. Clin Exp Allergy 2012;42:883–90.
66. Tan BK, Klingler AI, Poposki JA, et al. Heterogeneous inflammatory patterns in chronic rhinosinusitis without nasal polyps in Chicago, Illinois. J Allergy Clin Immunol 2017;139:699–703.e7.
67. Derycke L, Eyerich S, Van Crombruggen K, et al. Mixed T helper cell signatures in chronic rhinosinusitis with and without polyps. PLoS One 2014;9:e97581.
68. Gevaert P, Holtappels G, Johansson SG, et al. Organization of secondary lymphoid tissue and local IgE formation to Staphylococcus aureus enterotoxins in nasal polyp tissue. Allergy 2005;60:71–9.
69. Hulse KE, Norton JE, Suh L, et al. Chronic rhinosinusitis with nasal polyps is characterized by B-cell inflammation and EBV-induced protein 2 expression. J Allergy Clin Immunol 2013;131:1075–83, 83.
70. Gevaert P, Nouri-Aria KT, Wu H, et al. Local receptor revision and class switching to IgE in chronic rhinosinusitis with nasal polyps. Allergy 2013;68:55–63.
71. Tan BK, Li QZ, Suh L, et al. Evidence for intranasal antinuclear autoantibodies in patients with chronic rhinosinusitis with nasal polyps. J Allergy Clin Immunol 2011;128:1198–206.
72. Chen JB, James LK, Davies AM, et al. Antibodies and superantibodies in patients with chronic rhinosinusitis with nasal polyps. J Allergy Clin Immunol 2017;139:1195–204.
73. Takeda K, Sakakibara S, Yamashita K, et al. Allergic conversion of protective mucosal immunity against nasal bacteria in patients with chronic rhinosinusitis with nasal polyposis. J Allergy Clin Immunol 2018;143(3):1163–75.e15.
74. Steelant B, Seys SF, Boeckxstaens G, et al. Restoring airway epithelial barrier dysfunction: a new therapeutic challenge in allergic airway disease. Rhinology 2016;54:195–205.
75. Zhang N, Van Crombruggen K, Gevaert E, et al. Barrier function of the nasal mucosa in health and type-2 biased airway diseases. Allergy 2016;71:295–307.

76. Gon Y, Hashimoto S. Role of airway epithelial barrier dysfunction in pathogenesis of asthma. Allergol Int 2018;67:12–7.

77. Holgate ST. The sentinel role of the airway epithelium in asthma pathogenesis. Immunol Rev 2011;242:205–19.

78. Hamilos DL. Drivers of chronic rhinosinusitis: inflammation versus infection. J Allergy Clin Immunol 2015;136:1454–9.

79. von Eiff C, Becker K, Machka K, et al. Nasal carriage as a source of Staphylococcus aureus bacteremia. Study Group. N Engl J Med 2001;344:11–6.

80. Altunbulakli C, Costa R, Lan F, et al. Staphylococcus aureus enhances the tight junction barrier integrity in healthy nasal tissue, but not in nasal polyps. J Allergy Clin Immunol 2018;142:665–8.

81. Lan F, Zhang N, Holtappels G, et al. Staphylococcus aureus induces a mucosal type 2 immune response via epithelial cell-derived cytokines. Am J Respir Crit Care Med 2018;198:452–63.

82. Clark DW, Wenaas A, Citardi MJ, et al. Chronic rhinosinusitis with nasal polyps: elevated serum immunoglobulin E is associated with Staphylococcus aureus on culture. Int Forum Allergy Rhinol 2011;1:445–50.

83. Corriveau MN, Zhang N, Holtappels G, et al. Detection of Staphylococcus aureus in nasal tissue with peptide nucleic acid-fluorescence in situ hybridization. Am J Rhinol Allergy 2009;23:461–5.

84. Patou J, Gevaert P, Van Zele T, et al. Staphylococcus aureus enterotoxin B, protein A, and lipoteichoic acid stimulations in nasal polyps. J Allergy Clin Immunol 2008;121:110–5.

85. Zhang N, Holtappels G, Gevaert P, et al. Mucosal tissue polyclonal IgE is functional in response to allergen and SEB. Allergy 2011;66:141–8.

86. Tripathi A, Conley DB, Grammer LC, et al. Immunoglobulin E to staphylococcal and streptococcal toxins in patients with chronic sinusitis/nasal polyposis. Laryngoscope 2004;114:1822–6.

87. Van Zele T, Gevaert P, Watelet JB, et al. Staphylococcus aureus colonization and IgE antibody formation to enterotoxins is increased in nasal polyposis. J Allergy Clin Immunol 2004;114:981–3.

88. Kim YC, Won HK, Lee JW, et al. Staphylococcus aureus nasal colonization and asthma in adults: systematic review and meta-Analysis. J Allergy Clin Immunol Pract 2018;7(2):606–15.e9.

89. Bachert C, Gevaert P, Howarth P, et al. IgE to Staphylococcus aureus enterotoxins in serum is related to severity of asthma. J Allergy Clin Immunol 2003;111:1131–2.

90. Tanaka A, Suzuki S, Ohta S, et al. Association between specific IgE to Staphylococcus aureus enterotoxins A and B and asthma control. Ann Allergy Asthma Immunol 2015;115:191–7.

91. Bachert C, van Steen K, Zhang N, et al. Specific IgE against Staphylococcus aureus enterotoxins: an independent risk factor for asthma. J Allergy Clin Immunol 2012;130:376–81.

92. Kowalski ML, Cieslak M, Pérez-Novo CA, et al. Clinical and immunological determinants of severe/refractory asthma (SRA): association with Staphylococcal superantigen-specific IgE antibodies. Allergy 2011;66:32–8.

93. Biel MA, Brown CA, Levinson RM, et al. Evaluation of the microbiology of chronic maxillary sinusitis. Ann Otol Rhinol Laryngol 1998;107:942–5.

94. Chan J, Hadley J. The microbiology of chronic rhinosinusitis: results of a community surveillance study. Ear Nose Throat J 2001;80:143–5.

95. Boase S, Foreman A, Cleland E, et al. The microbiome of chronic rhinosinusitis: culture, molecular diagnostics and biofilm detection. BMC Infect Dis 2013;13: 210.
96. Cope EK, Goldberg AN, Pletcher SD, et al. Compositionally and functionally distinct sinus microbiota in chronic rhinosinusitis patients have immunological and clinically divergent consequences. Microbiome 2017;5:53.
97. Feazel LM, Robertson CE, Ramakrishnan VR, et al. Microbiome complexity and Staphylococcus aureus in chronic rhinosinusitis. Laryngoscope 2012;122: 467–72.
98. Ramakrishnan VR, Feazel LM, Abrass LJ, et al. Prevalence and abundance of Staphylococcus aureus in the middle meatus of patients with chronic rhinosinusitis, nasal polyps, and asthma. Int Forum Allergy Rhinol 2013;3:267–71.
99. Mahdavinia M, Engen PA, LoSavio PS, et al. The nasal microbiome in patients with chronic rhinosinusitis: Analyzing the effects of atopy and bacterial functional pathways in 111 patients. J Allergy Clin Immunol 2018;142:287–90.
100. Chalermwatanachai T, Vilchez-Vargas R, Holtappels G, et al. Chronic rhinosinusitis with nasal polyps is characterized by dysbacteriosis of the nasal microbiota. Sci Rep 2018;8:7926.
101. Yang HJ, LoSavio PS, Holtappels G, et al. Association of nasal microbiome and asthma control in patients with chronic rhinosinusitis. Clin Exp Allergy 2018; 48(12):1744–7.
102. Teo SM, Mok D, Pham K, et al. The infant nasopharyngeal microbiome impacts severity of lower respiratory infection and risk of asthma development. Cell Host Microbe 2015;17:704–15.
103. Navarro J, Rainisio M, Harms HK, et al. Factors associated with poor pulmonary function: cross-sectional analysis of data from the ERCF. European Epidemiologic Registry of Cystic Fibrosis. Eur Respir J 2001;18:298–305.
104. Mahdavinia M, Keshavarzian A, Tobin MC, et al. A comprehensive review of the nasal microbiome in chronic rhinosinusitis (CRS). Clin Exp Allergy 2016;46: 21–41.
105. Chalermwatanachai T, Velasquez LC, Bachert C. The microbiome of the upper airways: focus on chronic rhinosinusitis. World Allergy Organ J 2015;8:3.

Helminths and Asthma
Risk and Protection

Jamille Souza Fernandes, PhD[a,b], Luciana Santos Cardoso, PhD[c],
Paulo M. Pitrez, MD[d], Álvaro A. Cruz, MD[b],*

KEYWORDS

- Helminths • Asthma • Type 2 response • Regulatory molecules • Symptoms
- Anthelmintic treatment

KEY POINTS

- Type 2 response is the main response involved in both asthma and helminth infections. Some helminths may induce protection or worsen symptoms of asthma.
- The duration of infection, parasite load, and helminth species are factors that may influence the modulation of the immune response in asthma.
- Antigens derived from helminths with immunomodulatory properties may be new therapeutic candidates for asthma treatment or prevention.

INTRODUCTION

It is estimated that more than 1.5 billion people are infected by at least 1 species of geohelminths,[1] and more than 230 million people are infected by *Schistosoma* spp.[2] The prevalence of these infections is widely distributed, especially in less affluent communities.[1,3] In general, the symptoms are similar between species, including gastrointestinal manifestations, malnutrition, general malaise, and weakness. However, some species (*Necator americanus, Ancylostoma duodenale, Strongyloides stercoralis and Ascaris lumbricoides*) that bear a lung cycle can induce respiratory symptoms, such as cough, shortness of breath and wheezing.

Disclosure Statement: The authors declare that they have no conflict of interests to declare in relation to this article.
^a Centro das Ciências Biológicas e da Saúde, Universidade Federal do Oeste da Bahia, Rua Bertioga, n° 892, Morada Nobre, Barreiras, Bahia 47810-059, Brazil; ^b ProAR - Universidade Federal da Bahia, Salvador, Bahia, Brazil; ^c Departamento de Análises Clínicas e Toxicológicas, Faculdade de Farmácia, Universidade Federal da Bahia, Rua Barão de Jeremoabo 147, Salvador, Bahia 40170-115, Brazil; ^d Hospital Moinhos de Vento, Rua Ramiro Barcelos, 910, Bairro Moinhos De Vento, Porto Alegre, Rio Grande do Sul 90035-001, Brazil
* Corresponding author. ProAR - UFBA, Multicentro de Saúde Carlos Gomes, Rua Carlos Gomes, 270, Dois de Julho, 7ª andar, Salvador, Bahia 40060-330, Brazil.
E-mail address: cruz.proar@gmail.com

Asthma affects more than 350 million people worldwide.[4] It is heterogeneous and complex, with a variety of clinical phenotypes. Although asthma has been associated with increased urbanization, the mechanisms of this relationship are unclear.[5] The hygiene hypothesis proposed by Strachan in 1989[6] attempted to explain why asthma and other allergic diseases were increasing in industrialized countries. A possible explanation for this trend was a low early exposure to viral and bacterial antigens, which induce a T helper 1 (T_H1)-type response and result in lack of regulation of the immune system, predisposing to the type 2 immune response in newborns, which is associated with allergic diseases.[6,7] Several studies also have shown that helminth infection, by stimulating regulatory T cells (Tregs) and inducing the production of interleukin (IL)-10 regulatory cytokines, can prevent allergy in humans[8–10] and in animal models of asthma.[11–13] The aim of this review is to discuss how helminth exposure may influence asthma and the potential application of helminth molecules in the prevention or treatment of asthma.

IMMUNOPATHOLOGY OF ASTHMA AND HELMINTH INFECTIONS

Although helminths and asthma induce similar immune responses, they have different characteristics (**Fig. 1**). The type 2 immune response is the major pathway involved in the immunopathogenesis of most cases of asthma and immunity against helminths. This response is initiated after exposure to helminths and allergens by epithelial cells, which release IL-25, IL-33, and thymic stromal lymphopoietin

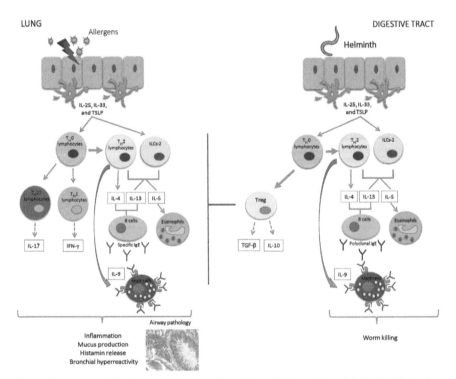

Fig. 1. Overview of the immune response in asthma (*left panel*) and helminth infections (*right panel*). Note that Tregs from helminth infections have the potential to suppress the asthmatic response in the lung.

(TSLP), inducing the cells of the innate and adaptive system to produce IL-4, IL-5, and IL-13. Different cell types, such as the innate lymphoid cells (ILCs2), basophils, eosinophils, mast cells, neutrophils, macrophages, and T lymphocytes and B lymphocytes are important in the immunopathogenesis of asthma and helminth infections. Thus, the interaction of these cells with cytokines stimulate IgE synthesis, and the release of inflammatory mediators, mucus production, and tissue remodeling. This interaction results in immunopathologic processes observed both in asthma and during a helminth infection.

It is known that the type 2 response is critical for the control of helminth infections and is the hallmark of allergic diseases.[14] In addition, T_H1 cell and T_H17 cell immune responses have been associated with asthma severity (reviewed by Lambrecht and Hammad[15]) and diseases caused by helminthic infections (reviewed by Cortes and colleagues[16] and Allen and colleagues[17]). In asthma, Kobayashi and colleagues[18] have shown that the administration of interferon (IFN)-γ increases airway hyperresponsiveness in an animal model and other studies have associated high levels of IL-17 with resistance to corticosteroid treatment in both an asthma animal model[19] and in humans.[20] As for helminth infections, the cytokines IFN-γ[21] and IL-17[22] have been associated with exacerbated granulomatous inflammation in *Schistosoma mansoni*–infected patients. On the other hand, these cytokines also amplify the type 2 response to a more pathologic state in both asthma and helminthic infections, especially with *S mansoni*. Randolph and colleagues[23] have observed that the transfer of T_H1 cells and T_H2 cells together caused more robust eosinophilic inflammation in comparison to a transfer of T_H2 cells alone in an animal model. Moreover, Irvin and colleagues[24] identified cells with IL-4$^+$CD4$^+$ T_H17 phenotype in humans, and the amount of IL-17 released by these cells in the bronchoalveolar lavage (BAL) was associated with bronchial hyperreactivity and airway obstruction. Finally, in an experimental model of schistosomiasis, the T_H17 response associated with severe hepatic granulomatous pathology was dependent on the expression of CD209a by dendritic cells,[25] with IL-4 or IL-13[26,27] responsible for positively regulating expression in these cells.

A type 2 response is the main pathway of the immunopathogenesis of both asthma and helminth infections (reviewed by Cruz and colleagues[28]); T_H1 and T_H17 responses are associated with severity, but the regulatory immune response is the great difference between them. In asthma, a reduction in Tregs has been reported in peripheral blood mononuclear cells (PBMCs) and BAL of patients with moderate to severe asthma.[29–31] In helminth infections, Tregs seem to protect the host from an excessive inflammatory response but also may limit the protective immunity and allow persistence of the parasite.[32] Because of this regulation induced by helminth infections, especially by *S mansoni*, several studies have shown that these infections can control or prevent inflammation observed in autoimmune and allergic diseases, such as asthma[8,10,12,13,33]

HELMINTH AND MODULATION OF THE IMMUNE RESPONSE IN ASTHMA

The life cycles of helminths are complex and, depending on the species, may include several intermediate hosts, different gateways, and migration within the host. In some species, such as *S mansoni*, *Strongyloides stercoralis*, *A lumbricoides*, and the hookworms, this migration can take them to the lungs. Consequently, helminths can influence lung immunopathology by direct damage to the lung tissue by the spread and deposition of eggs or release of immunomodulators.[34]

There are 4 factors that determine the modulatory effect of helminth infections on allergic diseases: (i) duration of infection, (ii) parasite load, (iii) host genetics and (iv) helminth species.[35]

Long-term infections seem more likely to induce immunomodulatory effects that suppresses allergic inflammation caused by parasitic and nonparasitic antigens. Layland and colleagues[36] observed that animals sensitized with ovalbumin (OVA) 5 weeks after infection by S mansoni showed a reduction in allergic inflammation of the airways, but this did not happen when the animals were sensitized 1 week after infection. In addition, heavy infections may induce immunomodulation, whereas mild infections induce the opposite effect. Studies in an experimental model of airway hyperresponsiveness have shown that administration of larvae of Strongyloides venezuelensis[37] or larvae of Heligmosomoides polygyrus[38] induced a protective effect. In humans, hookworm-infected asthmatic individuals with a high parasite load of 48 to 1458 eggs per gram of feces presented with less wheezing.[39] Host genetics may influence the ability to induce immunoregulatory mechanisms in the host. The authors' group described the variant (rs3024496, G allele) and other variants within the IL10 gene that were associated with decreased IL-10 production in peripheral blood leukocyte cultures stimulated with A lumbricoides antigens and a concomitant positive association with atopy and asthma.[40] Finally, different helminth species may exert different effects on the risk of developing allergic diseases, including asthma.[41] Cooper and colleagues[42] conducted a longitudinal study in an endemic region for geohelminths and showed that although children of mothers infected with geohelminths had more wheezing, children infected during the first 3 years of life had reduced risk of wheezing.

IMPACT OF HELMINTH INFECTIONS IN ASTHMA

There are several studies associating helminth infections with asthma symptoms, especially wheezing. These associations vary when comparing studies in animal models, populations of endemic areas, and clinical trials. Some species worsen or trigger asthma symptoms and others tend to prevent them. A systematic review[41] on the association of infections by intestinal parasites with asthma showed that infection with A lumbricoides associated with an increased prevalence of asthma. Studies conducted in urban areas in Brazil also have shown a positive association between infection by this parasite and bronchial hyperresponsiveness in children[43] and associated a high parasitic load of A lumbricoides with symptoms of asthma.[44] Nevertheless, another study did not observe an association of A lumbricoides infection with wheezing and asthma symptoms.[45] A possible explanation for the effects of A lumbricoides infection is its pulmonary cycle, because symptoms of asthma may be due to inflammation of the airways caused by migration of the larva or by an increased T_H2 inflammatory response. Other species, such as Toxocara spp[46,47] and Strongyloides spp, also are associated with asthma symptoms. The seroprevalence of Toxocara spp has been positively associated with high levels of total IgE and specific IgE to allergens, positive skin tests to allergens, and asthma prevalence and morbidity.[48] Other studies, meanwhile, have observed seropositivity to Toxocara spp associated with atopy but not with wheezing/asthma in children.[49,50] Regarding infection by Strongyloides spp, several studies have shown that Strongyloides stercoralis infection seems to mimic exacerbations of asthma, which may be refractory to the usual treatment of asthma.[51,52] Notwithstanding, a meta-analysis did not report any significant effect of Strongyloides stercoralis infection on the risk of asthma.[41] Other species of helminths, such as Trichuris trichiura[41,45] and Enterobius vermicularis,[41,53] do not seem to be risk factors for asthma.

What has motivated scientific interest are the species that can modulate the immune response in asthma and, consequently, prevent its symptoms. The most encouraging results were observed with *S mansoni* infection. Several observations in animal models have demonstrated that infection by this helminth seems to prevent against the development of allergies, including asthma.[12,54,55] In relation to studies of *S mansoni*–infected individuals, Medeiros and colleagues[56] have shown that asthmatic individuals living in an endemic area for *S mansoni* had a milder course of asthma at 1 year of follow-up compared with asthmatics not living in an endemic area of *S mansoni*. Additionally, it was shown that PBMCs from asthmatic individuals living in an endemic area and infected with *S mansoni* produced lower levels of IL-4 and IL-5 and higher levels of the regulatory cytokine IL-10.[9]

Hookworm infections also seem to protect against wheezing, asthma, and allergic diseases.[41] In a double-blind, placebo-controlled study, however, Feary and colleagues[57] showed that skin administration of 10 larvae of *N americanus* to asthmatic subjects did not result in improved bronchial hyperresponsiveness or other measures of asthma control. The infection was well tolerated, indicating that other studies that mimic natural infection are feasible and could be performed.

The impact of helminthic coinfections also has been studied. Alcântara-Neves and colleagues[33] found no association between the number of different current helminth infections with asthma, regardless of atopic status, in children in Latin America.

There are few studies reporting the capacity of helminthic infections to induce regulation when allergy is established. Wilson and colleagues[38] and Negrão-Corrêa and colleagues[37] observed that administration of *H polygyrus* and *Strongyloides venezuelensis*, respectively, after establishment of airway inflammation by OVA, were able to suppress allergic airways inflammation in the animal model. The first study noted that infection by *H polygyrus*, intestinal helminth of rodents, elicited Tregs that modulated allergen-induced pathology in vivo, with a reduction in numbers of eosinophils in the BAL. The second study observed that infection reduced airway hyperresponsiveness 48 hours after OVA challenge.

Overall, although the results of studies are highly variable, helminth infections appear to reduce asthma morbidity. Ponte and colleagues[58] performed a country-wide ecological study in Brazil and observed that populations exposed to infections by *S mansoni* and intestinal helminths had lower hospitalization rates due to asthma.

EFFECT OF ANTIHELMINTH TREATMENT ON ASTHMATICS

One way to investigate the impact of helminth infections on asthma is to treat the infections and observe any variation on asthma control. The reports vary depending on the species of helminth targeted by the treatment. A study conducted in asthmatics in Venezuela, where *A lumbricoides* and *T trichiura* infection were predominant, found that after treatment with albendazole subjects improved in symptoms of asthma.[59] Studies performed in children in an area endemic to geohelminths in Ecuador[60] and in a semiurban area in Uganda[61] found no association between anthelmintic treatment with asthma symptoms.

On the other hand, the authors' group conducted a double-blind, placebo-controlled study to assess the influence of anthelmintic treatments on asthma severity in individuals living in an area endemic for schistosomiasis and geohelminths. A clinical worsening of the disease was observed after 6 months and 12 months of treatment with antihelmintics.[62]

Overall, *S mansoni* is the parasite that consistently induces protection against development of allergies. Furthermore, several antigens of this parasite have been reported to prevent immune-mediated diseases of both T_H1 and T_H2 profiles.

IMMUNOMODULATORY MOLECULES OF HELMINTHS

Because helminth infections can modulate the exacerbated inflammatory response in asthma and consequently reduce its severity, researchers have investigated the potential for molecules derived from these parasites in exerting a regulatory function. A murine model of OVA-induced asthma showed that administration of excretory/ secretory products of the helminth *Fasciola hepatica* reduced the accumulation of mucus, eosinophils, and lymphocytes in the airways of allergen challenged mice.[63] Recombinant proteins of *S mansoni*, Sm22.6, Sm29, and PIII[13] or the antigen derived from schistosomula tegument (Smteg)[64] also were able to regulate the production of IL-5 and IL-13 and subsequent BAL eosinophilia in an experimental model of asthma. In addition, both studies observed that parasitic antigens are able to reduce lung inflammation and serum levels of OVA-specific IgE. The reduction observed in these inflammatory parameters was associated with increased levels of IL-10 and/or frequency of Tregs.[64] A study evaluating the effect of *Nipostrongilus brasiliensis* excretory-secretory products on the development of asthma in a murine model showed that reduction in IL-4 and IL-5 levels in the airways was independent of the presence of Toll-like receptors 2 and 4, IFN-γ, and, most importantly, IL-10.[65] In addition, Pitrez and colleagues[66] noted that different extracts of helminths inhibited lung allergic inflammation in mice and that IL-10 does not seem to play a central role in some helminth-host interactions. The investigators also point out that early exposure to helminth extracts could be a potential strategy to explore primary prevention in asthma.

Recently, the authors' group evaluated the in vitro effect of the *S mansoni* Sm29 antigen on activation/regulation markers and T_H2 cytokine production by T lymphocytes from subjects with severe asthma. In addition to increased production of IL-10 by PBMCs from these individuals, the authors noticed that the antigen induced an increase in the frequency of Treg lymphocytes (ie, $CD4^+CD25^{high}$ T cells) and a decrease in the frequency of activated T lymphocytes (ie, $CD4^+CD25^{low}$ and $CD4^+CD69^+$ T cells).[10] Moreover, the addition of the Sm29 antigen reduced the frequency of $CD4^+IL-5^+$ and $CD4^+IL-13^+$ T lymphocytes in the group of individuals with severe asthma, whereas the levels of IL-10 in PBMCs stimulated with the allergen *Der p*1 were increased.[10]

There are several mechanisms by which helminth-derived products can modulate the inflammatory response in asthma. Some of the main reports are summarized in **Table 1**. The induction of IL-10 seems to be the main helminth antigen–mediated mechanism of protection by modulating the exacerbated inflammatory response in asthma.[65] There are other regulatory mechanisms, however, induced by helminth-derived products, involving the induction of regulatory lymphocytes, dendritic cells, macrophages, and cytokines, such as transforming growth factor β and IL-35 (reviewed by Logan and colleagues[67]).

Clinical trials have shown helminth products can benefit individuals with inflammatory diseases.[68] In asthma, most studies have been conducted in vitro or in an experimental model. Thus, clinical trials with these helminths derived molecules are needed. The identification of a molecule with immunomodulatory properties against asthma may open a new phase in the therapy and control of this disease.

Table 1
Helminth antigens involved in the modulation of the inflammatory response in asthma

Helminth Antigen	Model of Asthma	Mechanisms of Protection	Reference
Fasciola hepatica excretory-secretory products	Murine model of OVA-induced asthma	↓ mucus, eosinophils, and lymphocytes in the airways	Finlay et al,[63] 2017
Recombinant proteins of *S mansoni* (Sm22.6, Sm29, and PIII) Antigen derived from Smteg	Murine model of OVA-induced asthma	↓ IL-5, IL-13 and eosinophils in BAL ↓ inflammatory cells in the lungs ↓ OVA-specific IgE ↑ IL-10 and Tregs	Cardoso et al,[13] 2010; Marinho et al,[64] 2016
Nipostrongilus brasiliensis excretory-secretory products	Murine model of OVA-induced asthma	↓ IL-5 in the airways independent of IL-10 production	Trujillo-Vargas et al,[65] 2007
Different extracts of helminths (*Angiostrongylus costaricensis*, *Angiostrongylus cantonensis*, and *A lumbricoides*)	Murine model of OVA-induced asthma	↓ lung allergic inflammation independent of IL-10 production	Pitrez et al,[66] 2015
Recombinant *S mansoni* Sm29 antigen	PBMC of asthmatic individuals	↑ IL-10 levels in supernatants ↑CD4$^+$CD25^{high} ↓CD4$^+$CD25^{low} and CD4$^+$CD69$^+$–activated cells ↓CD4$^+$IL-5$^+$ and CD4$^+$IL-13$^+$	de Almeida et al,[10] 2017

FUTURE CONSIDERATIONS AND SUMMARY

A protective role of helminthic infections on the development of allergic diseases, such as asthma, has been reported. Although infections by *S mansoni* have been consistently associated with protection, species of geohelminths have been related to increased symptoms of asthma. Helminth species and several other factors, such as host genetics, parasite load, coinfections, environment, poverty, timing, and duration of infection, may influence the modulation of the immune response and disease outcomes. The potential benefits of helminth infection in preventing asthma have been observed in animal models and in some observations of endemic area populations. Regarding the therapeutic potential of parasites for asthma, there are some positive observations in animal models and, to date, no significant results in clinical trials. Nonetheless, several experimental studies have demonstrated the regulatory potential of helminth antigens for asthma and, as such, deserve further investigation with the potential goal of primary prevention and/or novel treatment of asthma and allergies.

REFERENCES

1. WHO. Soil-transmitted helminth infections. Available at: http://www.who.int/news-room/fact-sheets/detail/soil-transmitted-helminth-infections. Accessed July 29, 2018.

2. Colley DG, Bustinduy AL, Secor WE, et al. Human schistosomiasis. Lancet 2014; 383(9936):2253–64.

3. WHO. Schistosomiasis. Available at: http://www.who.int/news-room/fact-sheets/detail/schistosomiasis. Accessed July 29, 2018.

4. GBD 2015 Disease and Injury Incidence and Prevalence Collaborators. Global, regional, and national incidence, prevalence, and years lived with disability for 310 diseases and injuries, 1990-2015: a systematic analysis for the Global Burden of Disease Study 2015. Lancet 2016;388(10053):1545–602.

5. WHO. Asthma. Available at: http://www.who.int/news-room/fact-sheets/detail/asthma. Accessed July 29, 2018.

6. Strachan DP. Hay fever, hygiene, and household size. BMJ 1989;299(6710): 1259–60.

7. Yazdanbakhsh M, Kremsner PG, van Ree R. Allergy, parasites, and the hygiene hypothesis. Science 2002;296(5567):490–4.

8. van den Biggelaar AH, van Ree R, Rodrigues LC, et al. Decreased atopy in children infected with Schistosoma haematobium: a role for parasite-induced interleukin-10. Lancet 2000;356(9243):1723–7.

9. Araujo MI, Hoppe B, Medeiros M Jr, et al. Impaired T helper 2 response to aeroallergen in helminth-infected patients with asthma. J Infect Dis 2004;190(10): 1797–803.

10. de Almeida T, Fernandes JS, Lopes DM, et al. Schistosoma mansoni antigens alter activation markers and cytokine profile in lymphocytes of patients with asthma. Acta Trop 2017;166:268–79.

11. Mangan NE, van Rooijen N, McKenzie AN, et al. Helminth-modified pulmonary immune response protects mice from allergen-induced airway hyperresponsiveness. J Immunol 2006;176(1):138–47.

12. Pacifico LG, Marinho FA, Fonseca CT, et al. Schistosoma mansoni antigens modulate experimental allergic asthma in a murine model: a major role for CD4+ CD25+ Foxp3+ T cells independent of interleukin-10. Infect Immun 2009;77(1):98–107.

13. Cardoso LS, Oliveira SC, Goes AM, et al. Schistosoma mansoni antigens modulate the allergic response in a murine model of ovalbumin-induced airway inflammation. Clin Exp Immunol 2010;160(2):266–74.

14. Allen JE, Maizels RM. Diversity and dialogue in immunity to helminths. Nat Rev Immunol 2011;11(6):375–88.

15. Lambrecht BN, Hammad H. The immunology of asthma. Nat Immunol 2015;16(1): 45–56.

16. Cortes A, Munoz-Antoli C, Esteban JG, et al. Th2 and Th1 responses: clear and hidden sides of immunity against intestinal helminths. Trends Parasitol 2017; 33(9):678–93.

17. Allen JE, Sutherland TE, Ruckerl D. IL-17 and neutrophils: unexpected players in the type 2 immune response. Curr Opin Immunol 2015;34:99–106.

18. Kobayashi M, Ashino S, Shiohama Y, et al. IFN-gamma elevates airway hyperresponsiveness via up-regulation of neurokinin A/neurokinin-2 receptor signaling in a severe asthma model. Eur J Immunol 2011;42(2):393–402.

19. McKinley L, Alcorn JF, Peterson A, et al. TH17 cells mediate steroid-resistant airway inflammation and airway hyperresponsiveness in mice. J Immunol 2008; 181(6):4089–97.

20. Nanzer AM, Chambers ES, Ryanna K, et al. Enhanced production of IL-17A in patients with severe asthma is inhibited by 1alpha,25-dihydroxyvitamin D3 in a

glucocorticoid-independent fashion. J Allergy Clin Immunol 2013;132(2):297–304 e293.

21. Stadecker MJ, Asahi H, Finger E, et al. The immunobiology of Th1 polarization in high-pathology schistosomiasis. Immunol Rev 2004;201:168–79.

22. Mbow M, Larkin BM, Meurs L, et al. T-helper 17 cells are associated with pathology in human schistosomiasis. J Infect Dis 2013;207(1):186–95.

23. Randolph DA, Stephens R, Carruthers CJ, et al. Cooperation between Th1 and Th2 cells in a murine model of eosinophilic airway inflammation. J Clin Invest 1999;104(8):1021–9.

24. Irvin C, Zafar I, Good J, et al. Increased frequency of dual-positive TH2/TH17 cells in bronchoalveolar lavage fluid characterizes a population of patients with severe asthma. J Allergy Clin Immunol 2014;134(5):1175–86.e7.

25. Ponichtera HE, Shainheit MG, Liu BC, et al. CD209a expression on dendritic cells is critical for the development of pathogenic Th17 cell responses in murine schistosomiasis. J Immunol 2014;192(10):4655–65.

26. Pello OM, De Pizzol M, Mirolo M, et al. Role of c-MYC in alternative activation of human macrophages and tumor-associated macrophage biology. Blood 2012; 119(2):411–21.

27. Relloso M, Puig-Kroger A, Pello OM, et al. DC-SIGN (CD209) expression is IL-4 dependent and is negatively regulated by IFN, TGF-beta, and anti-inflammatory agents. J Immunol 2002;168(6):2634–43.

28. Cruz AA, Cooper PJ, Figueiredo CA, et al. Global issues in allergy and immunology: Parasitic infections and allergy. J Allergy Clin Immunol 2017;140(5): 1217–28.

29. Mamessier E, Nieves A, Lorec AM, et al. T-cell activation during exacerbations: a longitudinal study in refractory asthma. Allergy 2008;63(9):1202–10.

30. Shi YH, Shi GC, Wan HY, et al. Coexistence of Th1/Th2 and Th17/Treg imbalances in patients with allergic asthma. Chin Med J (Engl) 2011;124(13):1951–6.

31. Hartl D, Koller B, Mehlhorn AT, et al. Quantitative and functional impairment of pulmonary CD4+CD25hi regulatory T cells in pediatric asthma. J Allergy Clin Immunol 2007;119(5):1258–66.

32. Sawant DV, Gravano DM, Vogel P, et al. Regulatory T cells limit induction of protective immunity and promote immune pathology following intestinal helminth infection. J Immunol 2014;192(6):2904–12.

33. Alcântara-Neves NM, de SGBG, Veiga RV, et al. Effects of helminth co-infections on atopy, asthma and cytokine production in children living in a poor urban area in Latin America. BMC Res Notes 2014;7:817.

34. Schwartz C, Hams E, Fallon PG. Helminth Modulation of Lung Inflammation. Trends Parasitol 2018;34(5):388–403.

35. Cooper PJ. Interactions between helminth parasites and allergy. Curr Opin Allergy Clin Immunol 2009;9(1):29–37.

36. Layland LE, Straubinger K, Ritter M, et al. Schistosoma mansoni-mediated suppression of allergic airway inflammation requires patency and Foxp3+ Treg cells. PLoS Negl Trop Dis 2013;7(8):e2379.

37. Negrão-Corrêa D, Silveira MR, Borges CM, et al. Changes in pulmonary function and parasite burden in rats infected with Strongyloides venezuelensis concomitant with induction of allergic airway inflammation. Infect Immun 2003;71(5): 2607–14.

38. Wilson MS, Taylor MD, Balic A, et al. Suppression of allergic airway inflammation by helminth-induced regulatory T cells. J Exp Med 2005;202(9):1199–212.

39. Scrivener S, Yemaneberhan H, Zebenigus M, et al. Independent effects of intestinal parasite infection and domestic allergen exposure on risk of wheeze in Ethiopia: a nested case-control study. Lancet 2001;358(9292):1493–9.

40. Figueiredo CA, Barreto ML, Alcantara-Neves NM, et al. Coassociations between IL10 polymorphisms, IL-10 production, helminth infection, and asthma/wheeze in an urban tropical population in Brazil. J Allergy Clin Immunol 2013;131(6): 1683–90.

41. Leonardi-Bee J, Pritchard D, Britton J. Asthma and current intestinal parasite infection: systematic review and meta-analysis. Am J Respir Crit Care Med 2006;174(5):514–23.

42. Cooper PJ, Chico ME, Vaca MG, et al. Effect of early-life geohelminth infections on the development of wheezing at 5 years of age. Am J Respir Crit Care Med 2018;197(3):364–72.

43. da Silva ER, Sly PD, de Pereira MU, et al. Intestinal helminth infestation is associated with increased bronchial responsiveness in children. Pediatr Pulmonol 2008;43(7):662–5.

44. Pereira MU, Sly PD, Pitrez PM, et al. Nonatopic asthma is associated with helminth infections and bronchiolitis in poor children. Eur Respir J 2007;29(6): 1154–60.

45. Alcantara-Neves NM, Veiga RV, Dattoli VC, et al. The effect of single and multiple infections on atopy and wheezing in children. J Allergy Clin Immunol 2012;129(2): 359–67, 367.e1-3.

46. Cooper PJ. Toxocara canis infection: an important and neglected environmental risk factor for asthma? Clin Exp Allergy 2008;38(4):551–3.

47. Ferreira MU, Rubinsky-Elefant G, de Castro TG, et al. Bottle feeding and exposure to Toxocara as risk factors for wheezing illness among under-five Amazonian children: a population-based cross-sectional study. J Trop Pediatr 2007;53(2): 119–24.

48. Buijs J, Borsboom G, Renting M, et al. Relationship between allergic manifestations and Toxocara seropositivity: a cross-sectional study among elementary school children. Eur Respir J 1997;10(7):1467–75.

49. Mendonca LR, Veiga RV, Dattoli VC, et al. Toxocara seropositivity, atopy and wheezing in children living in poor neighbourhoods in urban Latin American. PLoS Negl Trop Dis 2012;6(11):e1886.

50. Silva MB, Amor ALM, Santos LN, et al. Risk factors for Toxocara spp. seroprevalence and its association with atopy and asthma phenotypes in school-age children in a small town and semi-rural areas of Northeast Brazil. Acta Trop 2017;174: 158–64.

51. Altintop L, Cakar B, Hokelek M, et al. Strongyloides stercoralis hyperinfection in a patient with rheumatoid arthritis and bronchial asthma: a case report. Ann Clin Microbiol Antimicrob 2010;9:27.

52. Dunlap NE, Shin MS, Polt SS, et al. Strongyloidiasis manifested as asthma. South Med J 1984;77(1):77–8.

53. Bager P, Vinkel Hansen A, Wohlfahrt J, et al. Helminth infection does not reduce risk for chronic inflammatory disease in a population-based cohort study. Gastroenterology 2012;142(1):55–62.

54. Mo HM, Lei JH, Jiang ZW, et al. Schistosoma japonicum infection modulates the development of allergen-induced airway inflammation in mice. Parasitol Res 2008;103(5):1183–9.

55. Smits HH, Hammad H, van Nimwegen M, et al. Protective effect of Schistosoma mansoni infection on allergic airway inflammation depends on the intensity and chronicity of infection. J Allergy Clin Immunol 2007;120(4):932–40.

56. Medeiros M Jr, Figueiredo JP, Almeida MC, et al. Schistosoma mansoni infection is associated with a reduced course of asthma. J Allergy Clin Immunol 2003; 111(5):947–51.

57. Feary JR, Venn AJ, Mortimer K, et al. Experimental hookworm infection: a randomized placebo-controlled trial in asthma. Clin Exp Allergy 2010;40(2):299–306.

58. Ponte EV, Rasella D, Souza-Machado C, et al. Reduced asthma morbidity in endemic areas for helminth infections: a longitudinal ecological study in Brazil. J Asthma 2014;51(10):1022–7.

59. Lynch NR, Palenque M, Hagel I, et al. Clinical improvement of asthma after anthelminthic treatment in a tropical situation. Am J Respir Crit Care Med 1997; 156(1):50–4.

60. Endara P, Vaca M, Chico ME, et al. Long-term periodic anthelmintic treatments are associated with increased allergen skin reactivity. Clin Exp Allergy 2010; 40(11):1669–77.

61. Namara B, Nash S, Lule SA, et al. Effects of treating helminths during pregnancy and early childhood on risk of allergy-related outcomes: follow-up of a randomized controlled trial. Pediatr Allergy Immunol 2017;28(8):784–92.

62. Almeida MC, Lima GS, Cardoso LS, et al. The effect of antihelminthic treatment on subjects with asthma from an endemic area of schistosomiasis: a randomized, double-blinded, and placebo-controlled trial. J Parasitol Res 2012;2012:296856.

63. Finlay CM, Stefanska AM, Coleman MM, et al. Secreted products of Fasciola hepatica inhibit the induction of T cell responses that mediate allergy. Parasite Immunol 2017;39(10):1–6.

64. Marinho FV, Alves CC, de Souza SC, et al. Schistosoma mansoni tegument (Smteg) induces IL-10 and modulates experimental airway inflammation. PLoS One 2016;11(7):e0160118.

65. Trujillo-Vargas CM, Werner-Klein M, Wohlleben G, et al. Helminth-derived products inhibit the development of allergic responses in mice. Am J Respir Crit Care Med 2007;175(4):336–44.

66. Pitrez PM, Gualdi LP, Barbosa GL, et al. Effect of different helminth extracts on the development of asthma in mice: the influence of early-life exposure and the role of IL-10 response. Exp Parasitol 2015;156:95–103.

67. Logan J, Navarro S, Loukas A, et al. Helminth-induced regulatory T cells and suppression of allergic responses. Curr Opin Immunol 2018;54:1–6.

68. Rosche B, Wernecke KD, Ohlraun S, et al. Trichuris suis ova in relapsing-remitting multiple sclerosis and clinically isolated syndrome (TRIOMS): study protocol for a randomized controlled trial. Trials 2013;14:112.

Biologics for Asthma and Risk of Infection
Cause for Concern?

Joao Pedro Lopes, MD, Mauli Desai, MD*

KEYWORDS

- Biologics • Safety • Infection risk • T2 asthma

KEY POINTS

- Emerging biologics are efficacious in reducing asthma exacerbations in severe Type 2 asthma and have a favorable risk-benefit profile.
- No significant increase in severe infection (including from parasitic organisms) was seen in clinical trials, perhaps due to the redundancy of the immune system.
- Continued pharmacovigilance is needed to understand long-term safety of biologics.

INTRODUCTION

Rapid advancements have been seen in the treatment paradigm for asthma in the past decade with the approved use of several new biologic agents for severe asthma, and many more are in the pipeline. Biologics allow us to offer a tailored treatment approach to patients based on asthma endotype and phenotype, thereby moving us forward into the era of personalized medicine.[1] Biologic drugs are monoclonal antibodies that block specific targets along key inflammatory cascade pathways involved in the pathogenesis of asthma. Clinical trials of targeted monoclonal antibodies to immunoglobulin E (IgE), interleukin-5 (IL-5), IL-5 receptor, IL-4 receptor alpha, and thymic stromal lymphopoietin (TSLP) have shown promising results in patients with asthma refractory to conventional therapy, with reductions seen in asthma exacerbation rates compared with placebo and overall favorable safety profiles.

As these new biologics enter the market, it is essential to understand their risk-benefit profiles and maintain long-term pharmacovigilance. Targeted pathways in severe asthma are also ones implicated in host immune defense against pathogens;

Disclosure Statement: The authors have nothing to disclose.
Icahn School of Medicine at Mount Sinai, 1425 Madison Avenue, Box 1089, New York, NY 10029, USA
* Corresponding author.
E-mail address: mauli.desai@mssm.edu

therefore, theoretical concerns about infection risk arise when using these medications. In this article, the authors review available and experimental biologic therapies for severe asthma, with a focus on T2 inflammatory pathways, and discuss available clinical trial data on adverse drug effects with a specific focus on infection risk.

BIOLOGICS FOR ASTHMA: TYPE 2 PATHWAYS

Asthma is now broadly categorized as type 2 (T2) or non-type 2 (non-T2) asthma. The complex inflammatory cascade of T2 asthma involves T-helper cell type 2 (Th2) cells, B cells, eosinophils, epithelial cells, type 2 innate lymphoid (IL-C2) cells, IgE, interleukin signaling molecules (IL-4, IL-5, IL-13), and more. Asthma may also be classified as eosinophilic or noneosinophilic.[2] Biomarkers of T2 asthma in clinical use include serum IgE, blood eosinophil count, sputum eosinophil count, and fractional exhaled nitric oxide level.[3] Many patients with T2 asthma are inhaled corticosteroid (ICS) responsive; however, a subset of patients has severe asthma (about 5%–10% of asthmatics) refractory to conventional therapies. Targeted biologics are promising treatment options for these patients.

Non-T2 asthma is an entity characterized by the lack of elevation in T2 biomarkers. Much less is known about non-T2 asthma, which may represent a neutrophilic or paucicellular disease process. Many of these patients develop severe, refractory asthma, oftentimes less responsive to corticosteroids than T2 asthma. Currently, there are no approved biologics for non-T2 asthma, but this is an area of investigation. As well, the role of T2 biologic agents in non-T2 asthma, independent of eosinophil count, is being investigated.[4,5]

Blocking the inflammatory pathways of T2 asthma raises concerns about potential adverse effects given the other known and suspected functions of these pathways. Eosinophils and serum IgE, in particular, are thought to be important in host defense against pathogenic organisms, such as parasites and protozoa. This article takes a closer look at the important role of these molecules in host defense so as to better understand the potential implications of blocking these pathways.

THE ROLE OF IMMUNOGLOBULIN E IN INFECTION

IgE plays a key role in the pathogenesis of allergic diseases. In T2-driven immune responses, Th2 cells and IL-C2 cells secrete large quantities of IL-4 and IL-13, which in turn upregulate the production of allergen-specific IgE by plasma cells. Allergen-specific IgE binds to its high-affinity receptor on mast cells and basophils; subsequent binding of allergens to IgE leads to cross-linking of IgE receptors, cell degranulation, and release of potent mediators.

IgE is also thought to play an important role in the defense against parasitic diseases, in particular, those caused by helminths and some protozoa.[6,7] Parasitic infection is the most common cause of elevated IgE in developing countries.[8] Studies have shown the presence of elevated levels of IgE in subjects from tropical and subtropical areas endemic for helminth parasites,[7] such as sub-Saharan Africa, Brazil, and other developing regions (especially poor rural areas) of Africa, Asia, and Latin America.[9] Parasites that are known to cause elevated IgE include *Ascaris*, *Schistosoma*, and *Strongyloides*, as well as *Toxocara*, *Trichuris*, *Echinococcus*, hookworms, and filaria.[9–11] Increases can be seen in total, and parasite-specific IgE levels and an associated peripheral eosinophilia may be seen. Several studies have shown an important role of IgE in the immune response to specific species of parasites, such as the ability to opsonize *Schistosoma mansoni*,[12] generation of IgG1 parasite-specific antibodies, coating of parasitic larvae, and influence on mast cell response.[13,14]

Importantly, low or absent levels of IgE do not seem to predispose individuals to severe parasitic infections. This lack of susceptibility to parasitic infection is thought to be due to redundancy within the immune system, with multiple pathways and molecules involved in immune defense against parasitic infections. IgE-deficient animal models show strong immune defense mechanisms against parasites that are entirely independent of IgE.[15]

IgE elevation has been shown in some individuals infected with human immunodeficiency virus-1 (HIV-1), Epstein-Barr virus, and cytomegalovirus. However, the role of IgE is unclear, and it may, in fact, play a role suppressing immune responses to viruses.[16] One study showed binding of IgE to its high-affinity receptor was associated with decreased production of type I interferon upon exposure of plasmacytoid dendritic cells to viruses, such as influenza or rhinovirus.[17] In addition, a study by Tam and colleagues[18] hypothesizes that rhinovirus-specific IgE may also contribute to some asthma exacerbations. IgE is not thought to play an important role in bacterial infections because it does not activate the complement pathway or participate in opsonization.

THE ROLE OF EOSINOPHILS IN INFECTION

Eosinophils are white blood cells of the granulocytic lineage predominantly found in tissue. IL-5 is the critical driver of eosinophil development and differentiation.[11,19] Peripheral blood and tissue eosinophilia are commonly seen in helminth infections and occasionally in nonhelminth infections.[19] Parasitic infections are one of the most common causes of eosinophilia, especially in areas endemic for parasites. Common culprits, given their propensity to cause hypereosinophilia and their worldwide geographic distribution, include *Strongyloides*, *Toxocara*, *Trichinella*, and hookworms. Other parasites, such as filaria or *Schistosoma*, may infect patients who travel to endemic areas.[19]

Eosinophils are thought to play an important role in the host defense against helminth infections.[20] Several studies have shown an important role for eosinophils and IL-5 in killing specific helminths, such as *Strongyloides*,[21] *Angiostrongylus*,[22] and *Onchocerca*.[23] The mechanism involves eosinophil activation and local release of cytotoxic contents, such as toxic granules and reactive oxygen species.[19] The precise role of eosinophils is still controversial due to conflicting data from mouse models and the inherent limitations of such models, such as the use of pathogens that do not usually infect mice.

Eosinophilia has been described in particular viral infections, such as respiratory syncytial virus,[24] and HIV, and some fungal and bacterial infections.[25] However, acute infection with a virus or bacteria is more frequently associated with suppression, rather than elevation, of peripheral blood eosinophil counts.[26]

SAFETY PROFILES OF BIOLOGIC AGENTS FOR ASTHMA

Biologics currently available for use in severe asthma are ones that block the T2 pathway: one is a monoclonal antibody against IgE (omalizumab), three are agents that block the IL-5 pathway (mepolizumab, reslizumab, and benralizumab), and another, approved in October 2018, blocks the IL-4 and IL-13 pathways (dupilumab). Phase 3 studies were performed for anti-IL-13 agents (lebrikizumab[27] and tralokinumab[28]) but did not show consistent and robust results regarding their primary efficacy endpoints. Targeted biologics are also being developed for novel targets, such as TSLP. **Fig. 1** shows how these agents target the T2 pathway.

Clinical trials of approved biologics have shown them to be efficacious in reducing asthma exacerbations and generally well tolerated. Common adverse drug events, which typically occur in similar rates to placebo, are noted in both the drug package

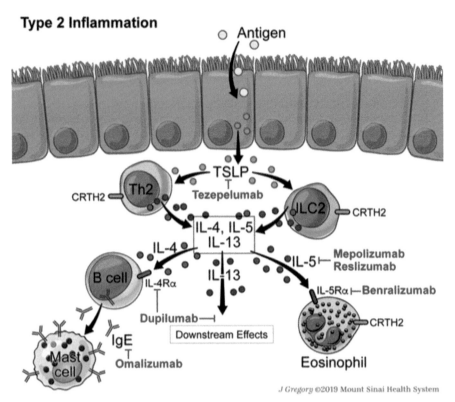

Fig. 1. Inflammatory pathways of asthma and targeted biologic therapeutics. (Printed with permission from ©Mount Sinai Health System.)

insert (as shown in **Table 1**) and the sentinel clinical trials (as shown in **Table 2**). There are black box warnings regarding anaphylaxis risk for omalizumab and reslizumab, and the package inserts for all contain statements regarding hypersensitivity reaction risk.

Omalizumab

Omalizumab is a recombinant monoclonal antibody that binds selectively to free IgE, inhibiting binding to its high-affinity FcεRI receptor expressed on the surface of basophils and mast cells.[29] It is administered as a subcutaneous injection, with dose and interval determined by weight and serum IgE level.[30] It was first approved by the Food and Drug Administration (FDA) in 2003 and is currently approved for use in patients aged 6 and older with moderate to severe persistent asthma, and a positive skin test or in vitro reactivity to a perennial aeroallergen, not controlled on ICSs.[31,32] Randomized, double-blind, placebo-controlled trials of omalizumab in subjects poorly controlled on combination controller therapy with ICS and long-acting beta-agonists have shown significant reductions in the rate of asthma exacerbations, in the range of 20% to 30%.[31,32]

Overall, long-term use of omalizumab has shown that it is well tolerated, but with potential adverse effects worth noting.[30,33] Omalizumab has a black box warning regarding anaphylaxis because of anaphylactic events reported in up to 0.2% of patients in premarketing and postmarketing surveillance.[30] Further review shows that the

Table 1
Biologic agents for asthma and adverse events: Information from package inserts

Drug	Mechanism of Action	Indication	Black Box Warning	Warnings and Precautions	Adverse Reactions
Omalizumab[30]	Anti-IgE	1. Moderate to severe persistent asthma in patients 6 y of age and older with a positive skin test or in vitro reactivity to a perennial aeroallergen and symptoms that are inadequately controlled with ICSs; 2. Chronic idiopathic urticaria in adults and adolescents 12 y of age and older who remain symptomatic despite H1 antihistamine treatment	Anaphylaxis	Malignancy, acute asthma symptoms, corticosteroid reduction, eosinophilic conditions, serum sickness symptoms	≥12 y: Arthralgia, pain, leg pain, fatigue, dizziness, fracture, arm pain, pruritus, dermatitis, earache 6–12 y: Nasopharyngitis, headache, pyrexia, upper abdominal pain, pharyngitis, otitis media, viral gastroenteritis, arthropod bites, epistaxis
Mepolizumab[42]	IL-5 antagonist	1. Add-on maintenance treatment of patients with severe asthma aged 12 y and older, and with an eosinophilic phenotype; 2. Adult patients with eosinophilic granulomatosis with polyangiitis		Hypersensitivity reactions, acute bronchospasm, herpes zoster infections, helminth infections	≥5%: Headache, injection site reactions, back pain, fatigue
Reslizumab[49]	IL-5 antagonist	Add-on maintenance treatment of patients with severe asthma aged 18 y and older and with an eosinophilic phenotype	Anaphylaxis	Malignancy, corticosteroid reduction, helminth infections	≥2%: Oropharyngeal pain

(continued on next page)

Table 1
(continued)

Drug	Mechanism of Action	Indication	Black Box Warning Warnings and Precautions	Adverse Reactions
Benralizumab[54]	IL-5 receptor alpha antagonist	Add-on maintenance treatment of patients with severe asthma aged 12 y and older and with an eosinophilic phenotype	Hypersensitivity reactions, corticosteroid reduction, helminth infections	≥5%: Headache, pharyngitis
Dupilumab[59]	IL-4 receptor alpha antagonist	1. Add-on maintenance treatment in patients with moderate to severe asthma aged 12 y and older with an eosinophilic phenotype or with oral corticosteroid-dependent asthma; 2. Adult patients with moderate to severe atopic dermatitis whose disease is not adequately controlled with topical prescription therapies or when those therapies are not advisable	Hypersensitivity reactions, conjunctivitis, and keratitis, eosinophilic conditions, corticosteroid reduction, helminth infections	≥1%: Injection site reactions, oropharyngeal pain, eosinophilia
Tezepelumab	TSLP antagonist	*No current approved indication*	*Not yet FDA approved for asthma*	

Table 2						
Biologic agents for asthma and adverse events: Information from clinical trials						
Drug	First Author, Year of Trial	Number of Subjects Randomized	Treatment Duration	Total Adverse Events	Commonly Reported Events (Similar to Placebo Unless Specified)	Infectious Adverse Event Rate Different from Placebo
Omalizumab	Humbert et al,[32] 2005	482	28 wk	Omalizumab subcutaneous (SC)[a] vs placebo (72.2% vs 75.5%)	Lower respiratory tract infections (RTI), nasopharyngitis, headache, sinusitis, injection site reactions,[b] influenza, upper RTI, cough	No
	Hanania et al,[31] 2011	850	48 wk	Omalizumab SC[a] vs placebo (80.4% vs 79.5%)	Bleeding, urticaria, injection site reaction, urticaria	No
Mepolizumab	Pavord et al,[45] 2012	621	52 wk	Mepolizumab intravenous (IV) 75 mg, 250 mg, or 750 mg q4w vs placebo (reported as similar)	Headache, nasopharyngitis, infusion-related reactions, hypersensitivity reactions	Herpes zoster (2 cases in mepolizumab vs 0 in placebo)
	Ortega et al,[44] 2014	576	32 wk	Mepolizumab IV 75 mg q4w, mepolizumab SC 100 mg q4w vs placebo (84%, 78% vs 83%)	Nasopharyngitis, headache, upper RTI, sinusitis, bronchitis, oropharyngeal pain, injection site reactions (for SC[b])	No
	Bel et al,[48] 2014	135	20 wk	Mepolizumab SC 100 mg q4w vs placebo (83% vs 91%)	Headache, nasopharyngitis, bronchitis, sinusitis, fatigue, nausea, arthralgia, oropharyngeal pain, upper RTI, adrenal insufficiency, pyrexia	No

(continued on next page)

Table 2
(continued)

Drug	First Author, Year of Trial	Number of Subjects Randomized	Treatment Duration	Total Adverse Events	Commonly Reported Events (Similar to Placebo Unless Specified)	Infectious Adverse Event Rate Different from Placebo
Reslizumab	Corren et al,[52] 2016	492	16 wk	Reslizumab[a] IV q4w vs placebo (55% vs 74%)	Asthma, upper RTI, sinusitis, bronchitis, nasopharyngitis, headache, urinary tract infection (UTI),[b] allergic rhinitis, influenza	Total infectious events higher in placebo (47%) vs reslizumab (31%); UTI (reslizumab 3% vs placebo 0%)
	Castro et al,[51] 2015	953	52 wk	Reslizumab[a] IV q4w vs placebo study 1 (80% vs 85%); study 2 (76% vs 87%)	Asthma worsening, upper RTI, nasopharyngitis, sinusitis, headache, influenza, nausea, bronchitis	No
Benralizumab	Bleecker et al,[56] 2016	1205	48 wk	Benralizumab SC 30 mg (q4w or q8w) vs placebo (72% vs 76%)	Worsening asthma, nasopharyngitis, upper RTI, headache, bronchitis, sinusitis, influenza, pharyngitis, rhinitis	No
	FitzGerald et al,[57] 2016	1306	56 wk	Benralizumab SC 30 mg (q4w or q8w) vs placebo (74% vs 78%)	Nasopharyngitis, asthma, bronchitis, upper RTI, headache, sinusitis, influenza, allergic rhinitis, hypertension	No
	Nair et al,[58] 2017	220	28 wk	Benralizumab SC 30 mg q4w, benralizumab SC 30 mg q8w (q4w in the initial 12 wk) vs placebo (68%, 75% vs 83%)	Nasopharyngitis, asthma, bronchitis, sinusitis, headache, upper RTI, rhinitis, influenza, back pain	Oral candidiasis (higher in placebo, 5% vs 0% for benralizumab)

Dupilumab	Castro et al,[60] 2018	1902	52 wk	Dupilumab SC (200 mg or 300 mg) q2w vs placebo (81% vs 83.1%)	Injection site reaction,[b] viral upper RTI, upper RTI, bronchitis, influenza, sinusitis, UTI, headache, allergic rhinitis	No
	Rabe et al,[61] 2018	210	24 wk	Dupilumab SC 300 mg q2w vs placebo (62% vs 64%)	Viral upper RTI, bronchitis, sinusitis, influenza, eosinophilia,[b] injection site reactions[b]	No
Tezepelumab[c]	Corren et al,[5] 2017	584	52 wk	Tezepelumab SC 70 mg q4w, tezepelumab SC 210 mg q4w, or tezepelumab SC q2w vs placebo (66.2%, 64.8%, 56.8% vs 62.2%)	Asthma exacerbation, nasopharyngitis, bronchitis, headache, injection site reactions	No

[a] Weight based.
[b] Significantly higher than placebo.
[c] Not yet FDA approved, phase 2 clinical trial.

actual incidence is likely less (around 0.09% of the patients).[34,35] Serum sickness-like reactions have been described after omalizumab administration[36] as well as fever, arthralgia, and rash.[30] There is also a warning about malignancy risk based on initial data; however, a prospective, observational cohort study published in 2014 compared 5007 asthmatics receiving omalizumab with 2829 asthmatics not receiving omalizumab and found no association between omalizumab and malignancy.[37] From this study,[37] the investigators noted an increased rate of cardiovascular and cerebrovascular events in the group on omalizumab, but a firm conclusion about cardiovascular risk could not be established because of study limitations.

A very low rate of helminth infection was identified in pivotal clinical trials of omalizumab.[33] The drug package insert recommends patients at high risk for geohelminth infections be monitored for such infections while on treatment.[30] In a randomized, double-blind, placebo-controlled trial published in 2007,[38] 137 subjects from several urban centers in Brazil, either actively infected with a geohelminth or at high risk for infection, were selected and treated with a broad-spectrum antihelminthic treatment. They were subsequently randomized to 52 weeks of treatment with omalizumab or placebo, with a primary study endpoint of rate of intestinal geohelminth infection. The study showed an insignificant trend toward an increased incidence of geohelminth infections in patients on omalizumab (50%) versus placebo (41%) (odds ratio = 1.47, confidence interval [CI] 0.74 to 2.95).[38] Of note, a study by Holgate and colleagues[33] did not mention an increase in helminth infections overall.

Pivotal clinical trials of omalizumab did not show a statistically significant increase in susceptibility to viral infections. In fact, a randomized controlled trial using omalizumab as preseasonal treatment analyzing 478 patients between the ages of 6 and 17 found considerable reduction of seasonal asthma exacerbations (omalizumab 11.3%, placebo 21.0%) in school children in the fall season, a time of peak incidence of respiratory viral infections.[17,39–41] The investigators hypothesize the mechanism for prevention of respiratory virus-induced asthma exacerbations associated with omalizumab use may be the restoration of virus-induced interferon alpha responses.[41]

Mepolizumab

Mepolizumab, a humanized monoclonal antibody against IL-5, received FDA approval in November 2015 and was the first anti-IL-5 agent to enter the market. The drug is approved for use as add-on therapy in patients aged 12 and older with severe asthma and an eosinophilic phenotype, as a once monthly subcutaneous injection at a dose of 100 mg every 4 weeks, and it is approved at higher doses for eosinophilic granulomatosis with polyangiitis.[42] Clinical trials of mepolizumab in patients with severe eosinophilic pneumonia have shown reductions in asthma exacerbations of about 50% and improved quality-of-life indices.[42–46] Treatment with mepolizumab has also been shown to have a steroid-sparing effect,[47,48] with a study by Bel and colleagues[48] showing a median reduction in oral corticosteroid use of 50% versus no reduction in the placebo group.

In pivotal clinical trials of mepolizumab, the drug was shown to have an acceptable side-effect profile. In the Dose Ranging Efficacy And safety with Mepolizumab (DREAM) trial, a dose-ranging efficacy study of mepolizumab in more than 600 subjects with severe eosinophilic asthma, the most frequently reported adverse events occurred at similar rates in the treatment and placebo arms: headache (mepolizumab 21%, placebo 17%) and nasopharyngitis (mepolizumab 19%–22%, placebo 15%). Three subjects died in the DREAM study (thought to be unrelated to treatment), and no life-threatening anaphylactic reactions were reported.[45] In subsequent trials of mepolizumab, headache and nasopharyngitis were the most commonly reported side effects. They were reported at similar rates in the treatment and placebo arms, as shown in **Table 2**.[44,48]

Analysis of the 3 randomized, placebo-controlled trials of mepolizumab[44,45,48] identified 2 cases of herpes zoster in the treatment arm and zero in the placebo group. Ongoing open-label extension studies of these clinical trials have identified several additional cases of herpes zoster infection in patients receiving mepolizumab. As such, the package insert recommends consideration of zoster vaccination in patients if clinically appropriate.[42] No mechanism for this association has been established. It is worth noting that an increase in herpes zoster infection risk has not been found in clinical trials of the other anti IL-5 agents reslizumab and benralizumab.

Despite theoretical concerns that anti-eosinophil treatment may expose a susceptibility to parasitic infection, no such increase in parasitic infection was noted in clinical trials of mepolizumab. Patients with active helminth infections were excluded from participation in clinical trials of mepolizumab. The recommendation on the package insert is to treat any patients with preexisting helminth infection before starting mepolizumab treatment and to discontinue mepolizumab in any patients who develop helminth infections not responding to antihelminth therapy while on mepolizumab.[42]

Reslizumab

Reslizumab received FDA approval in March 2016 as add-on therapy for the treatment of severe asthma with an eosinophilic phenotype, in patients aged 18 and older.[49] It is a humanized monoclonal antibody (IgG4 kappa) directed against IL-5 that is given every 4 weeks via the intravenous route at dosing determined by body weight (3.0 mg/kg). Two duplicate, multicenter randomized, placebo-controlled phase 3 clinical trials of reslizumab treatment of subjects with eosinophilic asthma (blood eosinophils >400/uL), inadequately controlled on medium to high doses of ICSs, showed significant reductions in the primary endpoint of asthma exacerbations compared with placebo, in the range of 40% to 50%.[50–52]

Pivotal clinical trials of reslizumab show that it is well tolerated; however, there was a 0.3% incidence of anaphylaxis seen, resulting in a black box warning regarding anaphylaxis.[49] In 2 duplicate phase 3 trials of reslizumab, Castro and colleagues[51] reported the most frequent adverse events were worsening of asthma symptoms, nasopharyngitis, upper respiratory tract infections, sinusitis, influenza, and headache; rates were similar between reslizumab and placebo groups. Similar adverse events were seen in the phase 3 trial by Corren and colleagues,[52] as shown in **Table 2**. Overall, there was a very low rate of serious infections reported with reslizumab.[53]

In aggregate, malignancies were seen more frequently in the treatment groups than in the placebo groups (0.6% vs 0.3%), but most of these were heterogeneous tumors diagnosed in the first 6 months of treatment; therefore, no causal relationship was found.[49,53]

Patients with known helminthic infections were excluded from trial participation. An increase in parasitic infections was not seen during clinical trials of reslizumab. The package insert recommendation is for any patient with preexisting helminth infection to be treated before starting reslizumab, and to discontinue the treatment in any patient who develops a helminth infection that does not respond appropriately to antihelminth therapy, until resolution of the infection.[49]

Benralizumab

Benralizumab blocks IL-5 receptor alpha, leading to near-complete depletion of eosinophils. It was approved by the FDA in late 2017 for patients 12 years of age or older, as add-on for maintenance treatment of patients with severe asthma with an eosinophilic phenotype.[54] It is administered as a subcutaneous injection; the first 3 doses are given every 4 weeks, followed by dosing every 8 weeks.

Benralizumab has been shown in clinical trials to reduce asthma exacerbations up to 50%, and it also has a steroid-sparing effect (75% reduction for benralizumab vs 25% for placebo).[55–58] In clinical trials, benralizumab has shown a favorable risk-benefit profile. Bleecker and colleagues,[56] comparing annual exacerbation rates of asthma in patients with severe asthma uncontrolled with high-dosage ICSs and long-acting B2-agonists, showed that both adverse events (benralizumab 72% vs placebo 76%) and serious adverse events (benralizumab 12% vs placebo 14%) were similar between groups, with the most frequently described adverse events listed as worsening asthma, nasopharyngitis, and upper respiratory infections. In a different trial published in the same year, FitzGerald and colleagues[57] showed that patients on benralizumab had a lower rate of adverse events when compared with placebo (74% vs 78%), as well as severe adverse events (10% vs 14%), with nasopharyngitis described as the most frequent adverse event, followed by asthma symptoms, bronchitis, upper respiratory infection, and headache.

Clinical trials of benralizumab excluded patients with helminth infections. The package insert recommendation is for any patient with preexisting helminth infection to be treated before starting benralizumab and to discontinue the treatment in any patient who develops a helminth infection who does not respond to antihelminth therapy until resolution of that infection.[54]

Dupilumab

Dupilumab is an IL-4 receptor alpha antagonist that blocks both IL-4 and IL-13 signaling. It was approved in 2018 as add-on maintenance treatment for patients with moderate to severe asthma, 12 years or older, with an eosinophilic phenotype or oral corticosteroid-dependent asthma.[59] It was previously approved for adult patients with moderate to severe atopic dermatitis when the disease is not controlled with conventional therapies, such as topical steroids.[59]

Two phase 3 trials were published in 2018; 1 study showed lower rates of asthma exacerbation, better asthma control, and lung function in patients with moderate to severe asthma, on dupilumab (at a dose of 200 or 300 mg), when compared with placebo.[60] In the second study, Rabe and colleagues[61] found that dupilumab use over a period of 24 weeks significantly reduced glucocorticoid requirements in the dupilumab arm (70%) versus placebo (42%).

In the first of those phase 3 trials, by Castro and colleagues,[60] the incidence of adverse events was similar in the dupilumab group (81%) and the placebo group (83.1%). The most frequently described adverse event was local injection site reaction, which occurred at a slightly higher rate in the dupilumab group. Other frequently described side effects were viral upper respiratory infection, bronchitis, influenza, sinusitis, urinary tract infection, and headache, with slightly lower rates in the dupilumab group compared with placebo. Eosinophilia was described at a higher rate in the dupilumab group than placebo (4.1% vs 0.6%). Eight patients were removed from the study (seven in the dupilumab group and one in the placebo group) due to eosinophilia-related adverse events. Two reported serious adverse events, with 1 patient having aggravation of preexisting hypereosinophilia (reporting fever, myalgias, arthralgias) and another patient developing chronic eosinophilic pneumonia.[60] In the second trial, Rabe and colleagues[61] described an incidence of adverse events similar between both groups (dupilumab 62% vs placebo 64%). The most frequently reported events described were similar. Of note, peripheral blood eosinophilia greater than

3000 cells per cubic millimeter was seen in the treatment group (14% vs 1% with placebo), but no clinical consequence of this was noted.[61]

Subjects with helminth infections were excluded from the clinical studies.[59] An increase in helminthic or viral infections was not seen.

Tezepelumab (Experimental Biologic for Asthma)

Many biologic therapies are in the pipeline for severe asthma. Tezepelumab is a human monoclonal antibody, undergoing phase 3 trials, that binds to TSLP, a cytokine produced in the epithelial cells as a response to proinflammatory stimuli. It is thought to have an important role in regulating barrier immunity, with downstream effects on many cells of the immune system, such as eosinophils, Th2 cells, and more. TSLP is thought to be a more upstream target of the T2 pathway; as such, blockade may potentially affect non-T2 pathways in asthmatic patients as well.[5]

In a phase 2 trial, lasting 52 weeks, in adults with uncontrolled asthma, tezepelumab was associated with a lower rate of clinically significant asthma exacerbations, irrespective of the eosinophil count. The most frequently described events were asthma symptoms, nasopharyngitis, bronchitis, and headache, all at similar levels in both groups. Infectious adverse events were very rare in the trial and occurred with similar rates in the tezepelumab group (2.5%) and placebo (2.7%).[5]

OTHER CONSIDERATIONS

This is an exciting time for the treatment of severe asthma because new biologic agents are being added to the treatment armamentarium. For many of these agents, phase 3 clinical trials show favorable risk-benefit profiles, without significantly higher risks of serious infections. It is important to note that for most of the newer drugs, there are only short-term data from clinical trials (most of which were 52 weeks or less). The exception is omalizumab, which has been approved for use in the United States since 2003, and long-term safety data are reassuring, as described in the real world omalizumab experience study by Holgate and colleagues.[33]

Despite concerns regarding the important role of IgE and eosinophils in infection, blockade of these pathways did not result in an increase in the rate or severity of helminthic infections in human subjects in clinical trials. The recommendation is that patients with active helminth infections should be successfully treated before starting treatment, as was done before enrollment in clinical trials.[30,42,49,54,59] There are no recommendations for screening for such infections before initiation of treatment, particularly in the United States where the incidence is relatively low. For individuals who travel to or spend a significant amount of time at areas endemic for geohelminth infections, that risk may be higher, and they may justify additional testing considerations.[33]

Many of the biologic agents described in the previous sections have been shown to have steroid-sparing effects, which is important to keep in mind when evaluating their risk profiles. Prolonged use of steroids and use of high doses of steroids are in themselves associated with an increased risk of infections.[62,63] It is hoped the steroid-sparing effects of biologic agents should reduce the risk of steroid-associated infections.

It is likely that new biologics will be seen entering the market. Novel potential therapeutic targets include IL-25 and IL-33, among others, and an antagonist to prostaglandin D2 receptor, fevipiprant, is under study.[64] With the arrival of all of the new biologics, it is vital for clinicians to remain abreast of the clinical indications for each as well as their unique adverse reaction profile.

SUMMARY

Although theoretical concerns exist regarding blocking pathways considered important in host defense against pathogens, clinical trial data do not show increased rates of parasitic, bacterial, or viral infections in the treatment versus placebo arms. It is reasonable to conclude that IgE and eosinophils are important in host defense against helminth infections, but it is unlikely that either alone is the sole critical pathway involved, given the redundancy of the immune response pathways.[10] Certain agents have special precautions, such as black box warnings for omalizumab and reslizumab, consideration for zoster vaccination with mepolizumab, and eosinophilia with dupilumab when used for eosinophilic asthma. Therefore, clinicians prescribing these agents should be familiar with each agent, potential adverse events, and their respective recommendations. Moving forward, pharmacovigilance with continued postmarking surveillance of suspected adverse events of new biologic agents will be of high importance in understanding long-term benefit-risk profiles.

REFERENCES

1. Darveaux J, Busse WW. Biologics in asthma—the next step toward personalized treatment. J Allergy Clin Immunol Pract 2015;3(2):152–60 [quiz: 161].
2. Carr TF, Zeki AA, Kraft M. Eosinophilic and noneosinophilic asthma. Am J Respir Crit Care Med 2018;197(1):22–37.
3. Zeiger RS, Schatz M, Li Q, et al. High blood eosinophil count is a risk factor for future asthma exacerbations in adult persistent asthma. J Allergy Clin Immunol Pract 2014;2(6):741–50.
4. Wenzel S, Castro M, Corren J, et al. Dupilumab efficacy and safety in adults with uncontrolled persistent asthma despite use of medium-to-high-dose inhaled corticosteroids plus a long-acting beta2 agonist: a randomised double-blind placebo-controlled pivotal phase 2b dose-ranging trial. Lancet 2016;388(10039): 31–44.
5. Corren J, Parnes JR, Wang L, et al. Tezepelumab in adults with uncontrolled asthma. N Engl J Med 2017;377(10):936–46.
6. Lynch NR, Hagel IA, Palenque ME, et al. Relationship between helminthic infection and IgE response in atopic and nonatopic children in a tropical environment. J Allergy Clin Immunol 1998;101(2 Pt 1):217–21.
7. Oettgen HC. Fifty years later: emerging functions of IgE antibodies in host defense, immune regulation, and allergic diseases. J Allergy Clin Immunol 2016; 137(6):1631–45.
8. Pien GC, Orange JS. Evaluation and clinical interpretation of hypergammaglobulinemia E: differentiating atopy from immunodeficiency. Ann Allergy Asthma Immunol 2008;100(4):392–5.
9. Hotez PJ, Brindley PJ, Bethony JM, et al. Helminth infections: the great neglected tropical diseases. J Clin Invest 2008;118(4):1311–21.
10. Cooper PJ, Ayre G, Martin C, et al. Geohelminth infections: a review of the role of IgE and assessment of potential risks of anti-IgE treatment. Allergy 2008;63(4): 409–17.
11. Stone KD, Prussin C, Metcalfe DD. IgE, mast cells, basophils, and eosinophils. J Allergy Clin Immunol 2010;125(2 Suppl 2):S73–80.
12. McSharry C, Xia Y, Holland CV, et al. Natural immunity to Ascaris lumbricoides associated with immunoglobulin E antibody to ABA-1 allergen and inflammation indicators in children. Infect Immun 1999;67(2):484–9.

13. King CL, Xianli J, Malhotra I, et al. Mice with a targeted deletion of the IgE gene have increased worm burdens and reduced granulomatous inflammation following primary infection with Schistosoma mansoni. J Immunol 1997;158(1):294–300.
14. Gurish MF, Bryce PJ, Tao H, et al. IgE enhances parasite clearance and regulates mast cell responses in mice infected with Trichinella spiralis. J Immunol 2004;172(2):1139–45.
15. Watanabe N, Katakura K, Kobayashi A, et al. Protective immunity and eosinophilia in IgE-deficient SJA/9 mice infected with Nippostrongylus brasiliensis and Trichinella spiralis. Proc Natl Acad Sci U S A 1988;85(12):4460–2.
16. Miguez-Burbano MJ, Shor-Posner G, Fletcher MA, et al. Immunoglobulin E levels in relationship to HIV-1 disease, route of infection, and vitamin E status. Allergy 1995;50(2):157–61.
17. Durrani SR, Montville DJ, Pratt AS, et al. Innate immune responses to rhinovirus are reduced by the high-affinity IgE receptor in allergic asthmatic children. J Allergy Clin Immunol 2012;130(2):489–95.
18. Tam JS, Jackson WT, Hunter D, et al. Rhinovirus specific IgE can be detected in human sera. J Allergy Clin Immunol 2013;132(5):1241–3.
19. Klion AD, Nutman TB. The role of eosinophils in host defense against helminth parasites. J Allergy Clin Immunol 2004;113(1):30–7.
20. Rothenberg ME, Hogan SP. The eosinophil. Annu Rev Immunol 2006;24:147–74.
21. Herbert DR, Lee JJ, Lee NA, et al. Role of IL-5 in innate and adaptive immunity to larval Strongyloides stercoralis in mice. J Immunol 2000;165(8):4544–51.
22. Sasaki O, Sugaya H, Ishida K, et al. Ablation of eosinophils with anti-IL-5 antibody enhances the survival of intracranial worms of Angiostrongylus cantonensis in the mouse. Parasite Immunol 1993;15(6):349–54.
23. Lange AM, Yutanawiboonchai W, Scott P, et al. IL-4- and IL-5-dependent protective immunity to Onchocerca volvulus infective larvae in BALB/cBYJ mice. J Immunol 1994;153(1):205–11.
24. Rosenberg HF, Dyer KD, Domachowske JB. Respiratory viruses and eosinophils: exploring the connections. Antiviral Res 2009;83(1):1–9.
25. Rosenberg HF, Dyer KD, Foster PS. Eosinophils: changing perspectives in health and disease. Nat Rev Immunol 2013;13(1):9–22.
26. Ravin KA, Loy M. The eosinophil in infection. Clin Rev Allergy Immunol 2016;50(2):214–27.
27. Korenblat P, Kerwin E, Leshchenko I, et al. Efficacy and safety of lebrikizumab in adult patients with mild-to-moderate asthma not receiving inhaled corticosteroids. Respir Med 2018;134:143–9.
28. Brightling CE, Chanez P, Leigh R, et al. Efficacy and safety of tralokinumab in patients with severe uncontrolled asthma: a randomised, double-blind, placebo-controlled, phase 2b trial. Lancet Respir Med 2015;3(9):692–701.
29. Chanez P, Contin-Bordes C, Garcia G, et al. Omalizumab-induced decrease of FcxiRI expression in patients with severe allergic asthma. Respir Med 2010;104(11):1608–17.
30. Food and Drug Administration. Xolair (omalizumab) label 2016. Available at: https://www.accessdata.fda.gov/drugsatfda_docs/label/2016/103976s5225lbl.pdf. Accessed September 1, 2018.
31. Hanania NA, Alpan O, Hamilos DL, et al. Omalizumab in severe allergic asthma inadequately controlled with standard therapy: a randomized trial. Ann Intern Med 2011;154(9):573–82.

32. Humbert M, Beasley R, Ayres J, et al. Benefits of omalizumab as add-on therapy in patients with severe persistent asthma who are inadequately controlled despite best available therapy (GINA 2002 step 4 treatment): INNOVATE. Allergy 2005; 60(3):309–16.

33. Holgate S, Buhl R, Bousquet J, et al. The use of omalizumab in the treatment of severe allergic asthma: a clinical experience update. Respir Med 2009;103(8): 1098–113.

34. Cox L, Platts-Mills TA, Finegold I, et al. American Academy of Allergy, Asthma & Immunology/American College of Allergy, Asthma and Immunology Joint Task Force Report on omalizumab-associated anaphylaxis. J Allergy Clin Immunol 2007;120(6):1373–7.

35. Cox L, Lieberman P, Wallace D, et al. American Academy of Allergy, Asthma & Immunology/American College of Allergy, Asthma & Immunology Omalizumab-Associated Anaphylaxis Joint Task Force follow-up report. J Allergy Clin Immunol 2011;128(1):210–2.

36. Dreyfus DH, Randolph CC. Characterization of an anaphylactoid reaction to omalizumab. Ann Allergy Asthma Immunol 2006;96(4):624–7.

37. Long A, Rahmaoui A, Rothman KJ, et al. Incidence of malignancy in patients with moderate-to-severe asthma treated with or without omalizumab. J Allergy Clin Immunol 2014;134(3):560–7.e4.

38. Cruz AA, Lima F, Sarinho E, et al. Safety of anti-immunoglobulin E therapy with omalizumab in allergic patients at risk of geohelminth infection. Clin Exp Allergy 2007;37(2):197–207.

39. Busse WW, Morgan WJ, Gergen PJ, et al. Randomized trial of omalizumab (anti-IgE) for asthma in inner-city children. N Engl J Med 2011;364(11):1005–15.

40. Gill MA, Bajwa G, George TA, et al. Counterregulation between the FcepsilonRI pathway and antiviral responses in human plasmacytoid dendritic cells. J Immunol 2010;184(11):5999–6006.

41. Teach SJ, Gill MA, Togias A, et al. Preseasonal treatment with either omalizumab or an inhaled corticosteroid boost to prevent fall asthma exacerbations. J Allergy Clin Immunol 2015;136(6):1476–85.

42. Food and Drug Administration. Nucala (mepolizumab) label 2017. Available at: https://www.accessdata.fda.gov/drugsatfda_docs/label/2017/125526s004lbl.pdf. Accessed September 1, 2018.

43. Haldar P, Brightling CE, Hargadon B, et al. Mepolizumab and exacerbations of refractory eosinophilic asthma. N Engl J Med 2009;360(10):973–84.

44. Ortega HG, Liu MC, Pavord ID, et al. Mepolizumab treatment in patients with severe eosinophilic asthma. N Engl J Med 2014;371(13):1198–207.

45. Pavord ID, Korn S, Howarth P, et al. Mepolizumab for severe eosinophilic asthma (DREAM): a multicentre, double-blind, placebo-controlled trial. Lancet 2012; 380(9842):651–9.

46. Farne HA, Wilson A, Powell C, et al. Anti-IL5 therapies for asthma. Cochrane Database Syst Rev 2017;(9):CD010834.

47. Nair P, Pizzichini MM, Kjarsgaard M, et al. Mepolizumab for prednisone-dependent asthma with sputum eosinophilia. N Engl J Med 2009;360(10): 985–93.

48. Bel EH, Wenzel SE, Thompson PJ, et al. Oral glucocorticoid-sparing effect of mepolizumab in eosinophilic asthma. N Engl J Med 2014;371(13):1189–97.

49. Food and Drug Administration. Cinqair (reslizumab) label 2016. Available at: https://www.accessdata.fda.gov/drugsatfda_docs/label/2016/761033lbl.pdf. Accessed September 1, 2018.

50. Castro M, Mathur S, Hargreave F, et al. Reslizumab for poorly controlled, eosinophilic asthma: a randomized, placebo-controlled study. Am J Respir Crit Care Med 2011;184(10):1125–32.
51. Castro M, Zangrilli J, Wechsler ME, et al. Reslizumab for inadequately controlled asthma with elevated blood eosinophil counts: results from two multicentre, parallel, double-blind, randomised, placebo-controlled, phase 3 trials. Lancet Respir Med 2015;3(5):355–66.
52. Corren J, Weinstein S, Janka L, et al. Phase 3 study of reslizumab in patients with poorly controlled asthma: effects across a broad range of eosinophil counts. Chest 2016;150(4):799–810.
53. Murphy K, Jacobs J, Bjermer L, et al. Long-term safety and efficacy of reslizumab in patients with eosinophilic asthma. J Allergy Clin Immunol Pract 2017;5(6):1572–81.e3.
54. Food and Drug Administration. Fasenra (benralizumab) label 2017. Available at: https://www.accessdata.fda.gov/drugsatfda_docs/label/2017/761070s000lbl.pdf. Accessed September 1, 2018.
55. Castro M, Wenzel SE, Bleecker ER, et al. Benralizumab, an anti-interleukin 5 receptor alpha monoclonal antibody, versus placebo for uncontrolled eosinophilic asthma: a phase 2b randomised dose-ranging study. Lancet Respir Med 2014;2(11):879–90.
56. Bleecker ER, FitzGerald JM, Chanez P, et al. Efficacy and safety of benralizumab for patients with severe asthma uncontrolled with high-dosage inhaled corticosteroids and long-acting beta2-agonists (SIROCCO): a randomised, multicentre, placebo-controlled phase 3 trial. Lancet 2016;388(10056):2115–27.
57. FitzGerald JM, Bleecker ER, Nair P, et al. Benralizumab, an anti-interleukin-5 receptor alpha monoclonal antibody, as add-on treatment for patients with severe, uncontrolled, eosinophilic asthma (CALIMA): a randomised, double-blind, placebo-controlled phase 3 trial. Lancet 2016;388(10056):2128–41.
58. Nair P, Wenzel S, Rabe KF, et al. Oral glucocorticoid-sparing effect of benralizumab in severe asthma. N Engl J Med 2017;376(25):2448–58.
59. Food and Drug Administration. Dupixent (dupilumab) label 2018. Available at: https://www.accessdata.fda.gov/drugsatfda_docs/label/2017/761055lbl.pdf. Accessed October 25, 2018.
60. Castro M, Corren J, Pavord ID, et al. Dupilumab efficacy and safety in moderate-to-severe uncontrolled asthma. N Engl J Med 2018;378(26):2486–96.
61. Rabe KF, Nair P, Brusselle G, et al. Efficacy and safety of dupilumab in glucocorticoid-dependent severe asthma. N Engl J Med 2018;378(26):2475–85.
62. Rostaing L, Malvezzi P. Steroid-based therapy and risk of infectious complications. PLoS Med 2016;13(5):e1002025.
63. Dixon WG, Kezouh A, Bernatsky S, et al. The influence of systemic glucocorticoid therapy upon the risk of non-serious infection in older patients with rheumatoid arthritis: a nested case-control study. Ann Rheum Dis 2011;70(6):956–60.
64. Gonem S, Berair R, Singapuri A, et al. Fevipiprant, a prostaglandin D2 receptor 2 antagonist, in patients with persistent eosinophilic asthma: a single-centre, randomised, double-blind, parallel-group, placebo-controlled trial. Lancet Respir Med 2016;4(9):699–707.

Moving?

Make sure your subscription moves with you!

To notify us of your new address, find your **Clinics Account Number** (located on your mailing label above your name), and contact customer service at:

Email: journalscustomerservice-usa@elsevier.com

800-654-2452 (subscribers in the U.S. & Canada)
314-447-8871 (subscribers outside of the U.S. & Canada)

Fax number: 314-447-8029

Elsevier Health Sciences Division
Subscription Customer Service
3251 Riverport Lane
Maryland Heights, MO 63043

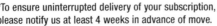
*To ensure uninterrupted delivery of your subscription, please notify us at least 4 weeks in advance of move.

ELSEVIER

Printed and bound by CPI Group (UK) Ltd, Croydon, CR0 4YY

03/10/2024

01040482-0012